How to Dress

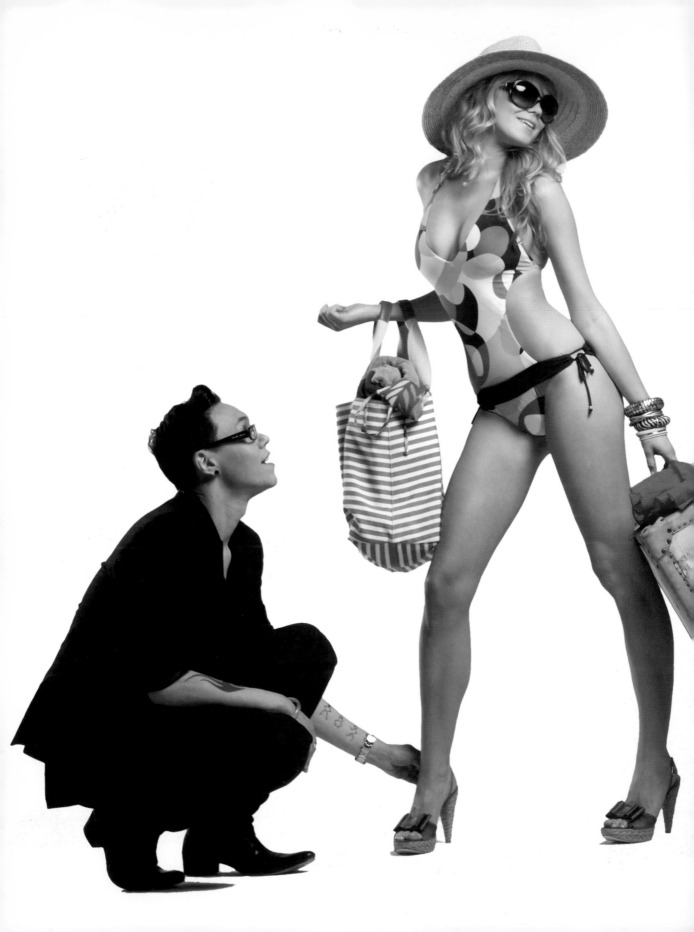

GOK·WAN

How to Dress

Your complete style guide for every occasion

HarperCollins*Publishers*

HarperCollins*Publishers*
77–85 Fulham Palace Road,
Hammersmith, London W6 8JB
www.harpercollins.co.uk

Published by HarperCollins*Publishers* 2008
This edition 2009
1

Edited by Angela Buttolph
Photographs © Roger Charity
Photographs pp. 10, 37, 67, 75, 93, 121, 155, 187, 213, 224, 237 © Adam Lawrence

A CIP catalogue record for this book
is available from the British Library

ISBN 978-0-00-729900-3

Printed in Italy by
Rotolito Lombarda, Milan, Italy

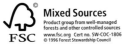

CONTENTS

Introduction 8

Basics 13

Underwear 39

Workwear 69

Going Out 95

Holidays 123

Weddings 157

Mums 189

Beauty 215

Shopping 227
Acknowledgements 248
Directory 250

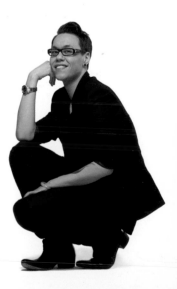

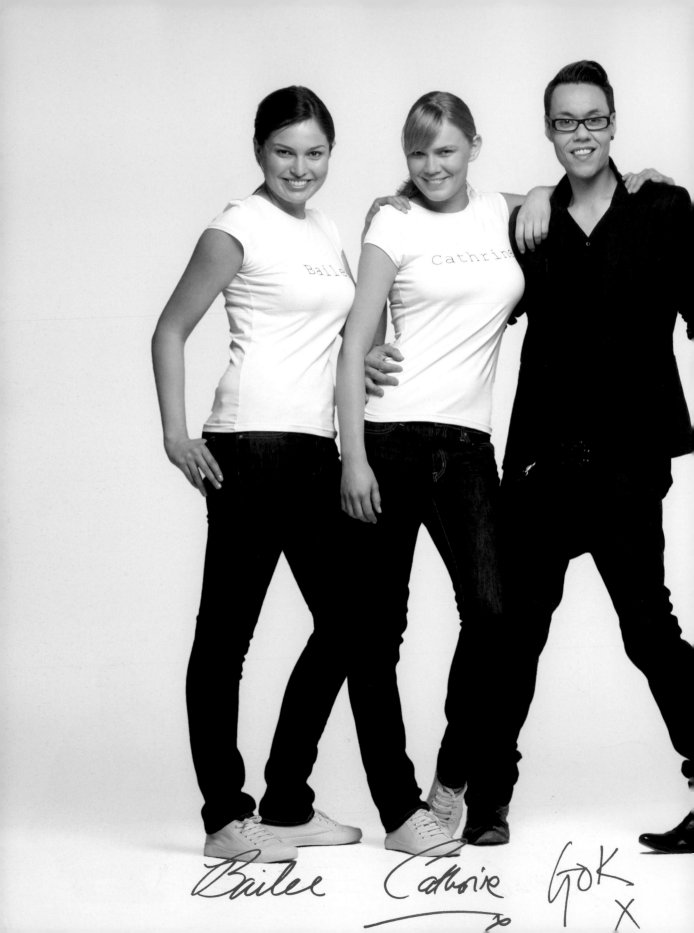

Bailee   Cathrine   GOK
                        x

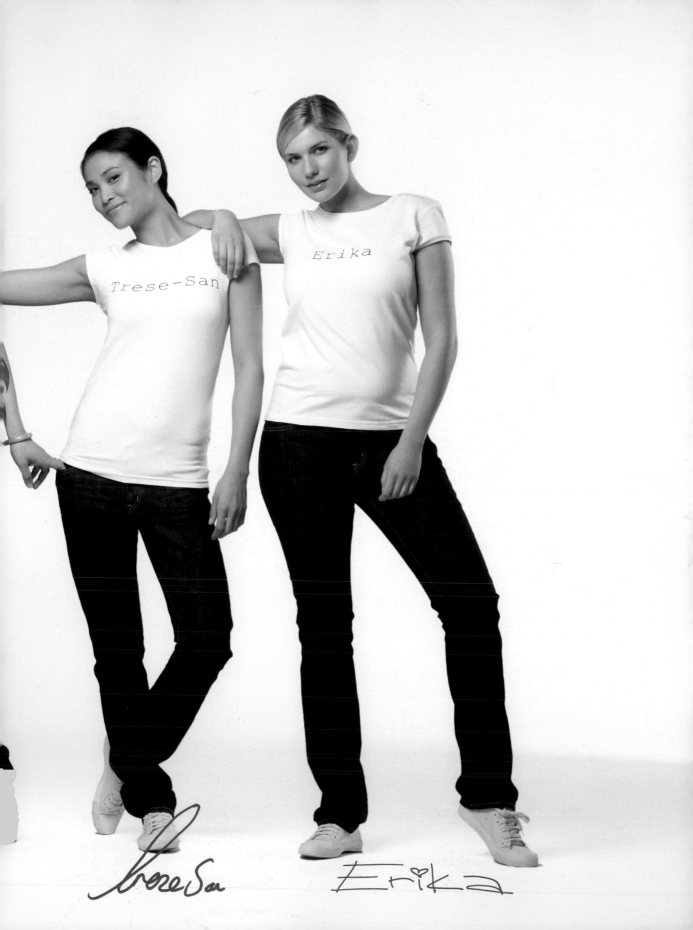

Gorgeous girl,

Don't think I don't know you dream of having the style of Sophia Loren, the boldness of Nicole Kidman and the effort-less sophistication of Jennifer Aniston.

Honey, let me let you into a little secret: nearly all celebs have stylists. A huge team of people behind them making them look that good.

How can you ever compete? Well, from now on, I'm going to be your personal stylist. Let me advise you on how to get dressed, and how not to get stressed.

I am so proud of British fashion. We have the best high street in the world. Whether you have £5 or £500 to spend, there are great clothes out there for you. But, there's a national epidemic; people don't know how to put outfits together! Finding clothes you love is just the start, because then, you have to get dressed …

Let me tell you, every woman gets stuck in a style rut once in a while. And every woman sometimes suffers from wardrobe-phobia. But life is too short not to enjoy shopping and dressing! There isn't a single person in the world that doesn't have the right to feel good about their personal appearance.

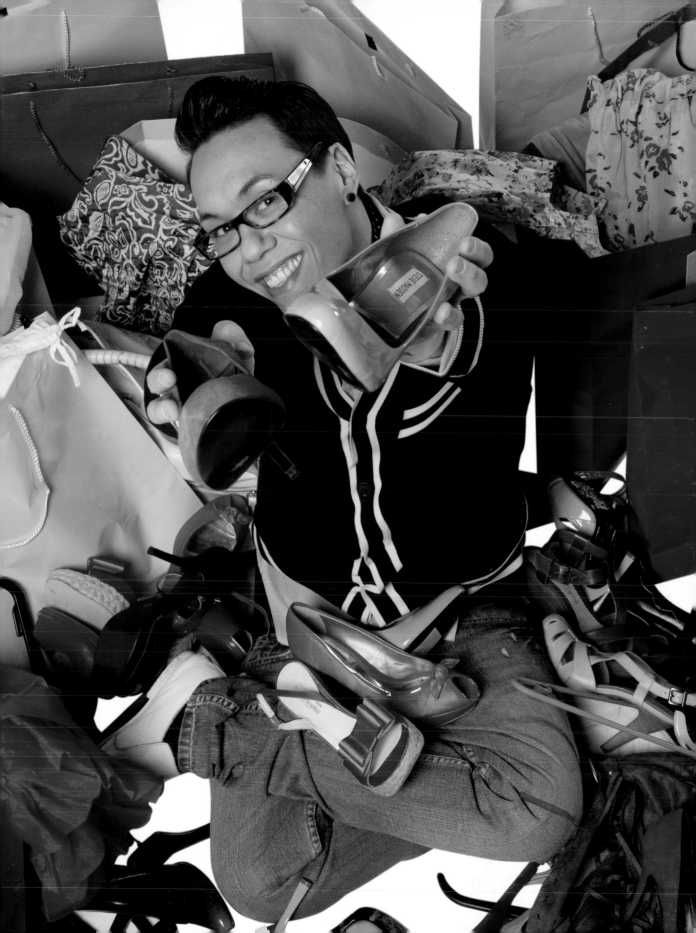

There is a knack to putting together a great outfit. Part of it is the way you combine your clothes and accessories, and part of it is knowing where to wear that outfit (or knowing the perfect outfit to wear to each event). And I'm going to show you how, because when someone comes up and says 'I love your outfit', it's the best compliment in the world, so let's make that happen more often.

Life is a series of celebrations (thank goodness!). Sooner or later, everyone's got an event to go to, and unless you're going to move into a naturist site in Bournemouth, you'll have to get dressed up!

I want to give you your very own one-to-one personal styling session, finding you the perfect clothes for every occasion.

By the time you've finished this book, you're going to feel like you've had a day of loving clothes, embracing your personal style and rejoicing in accessories. You'll be able to pull some new outfits out from every section of this book (and many more from your existing wardrobe!).

This book is going to buy you time. You're so busy with the kids or with work, why add to your hectic schedule by worrying about what to wear? Let this book take the worry away. And inspire you!

What this book will also do is give you more va-va-voom. You're going to feel like you want to mingle with people from work, enjoy the pregnancy and feel beautiful, go to that wedding and meet the man of your dreams, or go on holiday and take time out to relax. And you'll enjoy getting ready as much as you do going out.

I love clothes and putting them together, so this is going to be fun!

One last thing. What are you wearing right now?

Girlfriend, I want you to go and get your highest stilettos. Put 'em on, and turn the page, cos here's where we start the styling ...

love,

Gok
x

BASICS

Effortless, essential and eternally elegant

- Layering without adding bulk
- How to wear your favourite summer pieces all year round
- Sexy looks that don't flash too much flesh

Gorgeous lady, I was thinking about this chapter the other night and wondered — how does a woman get her wardrobe right if she doesn't get her basics right? The average woman (although, honey, you are far from average) has a wardrobe made up of four main areas: jeans, jersey, outerwear and knitwear. Sounds simple, right? Wrong! But honey, don't worry, because Uncle Gok is here to guide you through the Wardrobe Warzone that can be your basic pieces.

The whole point of basics is that they work like a wardrobe undercoat. They are the things that enable you to update your look every season without buying a whole new set of clothes. Some basics — like T-shirts and jeans — are the kind of things you'll wear every day (or when you don't have time to think about what to put on), whereas other pieces, like a leather jacket or a classic trench, are things it's good to invest in, as they'll work for years to come with that must-have new dress or pair of trousers.

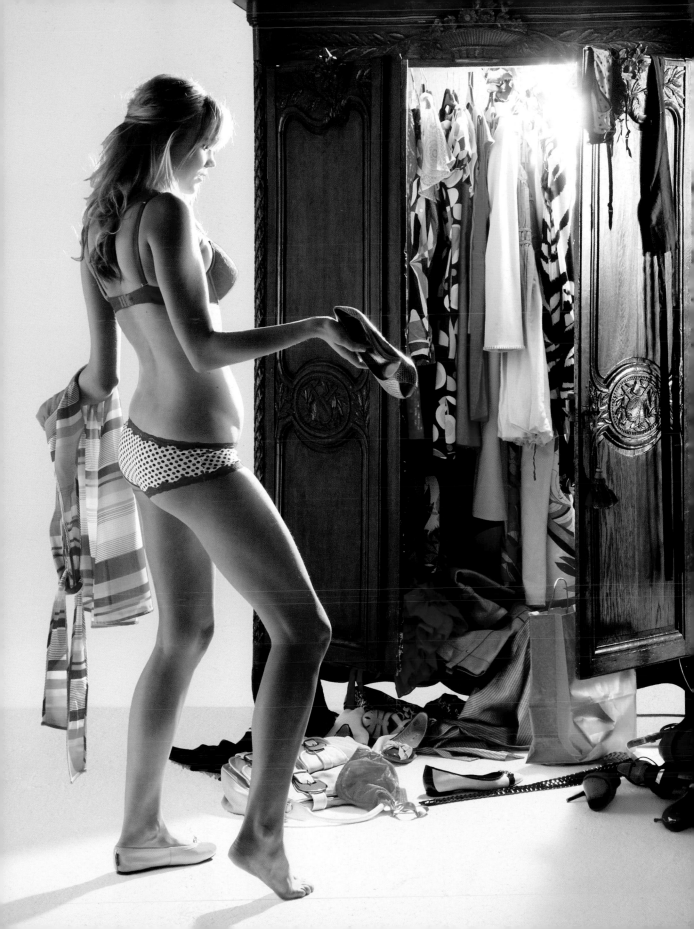

Either way, it makes sense to think about quality when you're shopping for basics. Gap does the best cotton on the high street, and American Apparel has more sexy jersey pieces than you'll need in a lifetime. Specialist jeans shops like Levi's, Lee and Wrangler will have more fits and sizes than high street stores, so it pays to go off the beaten track when you're doing your basic buying.

Top of most women's list of Shopping Nightmares is buying jeans. Lady, you are not alone! There's so much to choose from, so many shapes and washes and fabrics that it's a style minefield. Well, I'm going to take you through the three key shapes out there at the moment – skinny, boot-cut and wide-legged – so we can find the perfect pair for you to flatter that fabulous figure of yours.

Jersey isn't much easier than denim when it comes to wardrobe staples. In fact, there's so much out there on the high street that it would be possible to wear nothing but jersey every day, with shops like Agnès b and Nicole Farhi specializing in it.

The key to jersey basics is to embrace the fabric itself. It's a great, heavy, slinky fabric that skims rather than clings, and can look super-sexy or dressed-down casual depending on how you wear it. Have a look at my tips in this chapter to see the best ways for you to wear jersey, and the best simple pieces for your basics wardrobe.

Knitwear is another minefield simply because it (totally unfairly!) has a frumpy image. But, my gorgeous, by breaking those old rules and mixing chunky knits and summer dresses, or winter warmers and skinny knits, you can add texture to your outfit and personality to your look.

Finally, with coats and jackets we'll look at the key shapes and fabrics for you to keep in your wardrobe and update season after season. From a classic bomber jacket to a woollen winter coat, these are pieces it's good to invest in as they'll be there to take you through several nights out, a couple of weddings, a handful of day trips and a weekend away! Just like me, girlfriend, they're on hand to help keep you looking stylish and fabulous whatever the occasion.

Lots of my girls feel nervous about layering their clothes, so I've chosen some looks where we've mixed those basics up with some funkier pieces, to show you how to give new life to a fabulous summer dress (layer it under a skinny-fit polo) or a classic winter coat by belting it differently.

In fact, layering is one of the best ways to breathe new life into your wardrobe, and there are just a few simple rules to stick to when you're trying it at home:

- Keep base layers in a thin fabric so that you don't overheat; it's tricky to remove the underneath layer once you're out and about!
- Keep top layers low cut and short sleeved, so you can see the layer underneath, to make a confident style statement.
- If you're mixing pattern with plain colours, then keep the pattern on top so it doesn't get lost.

So, girlfriend, let's have a bash at those basics!

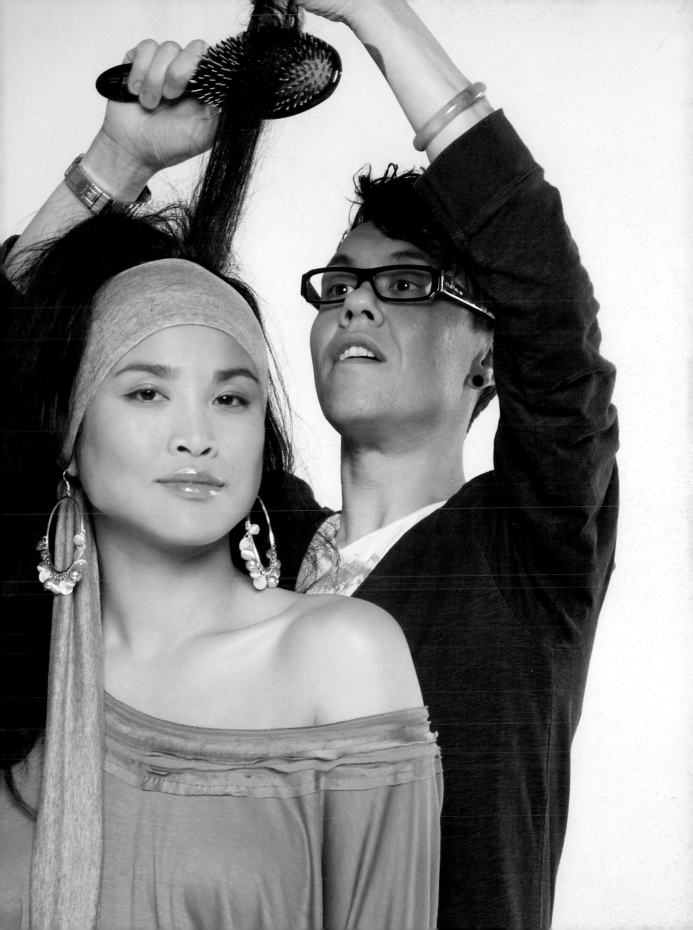

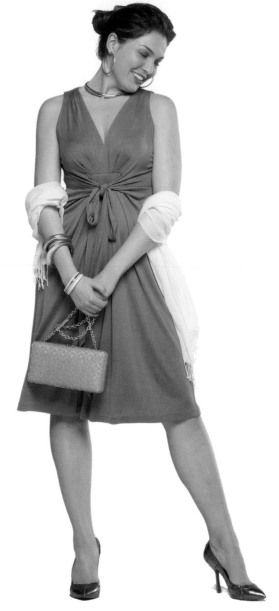

Neutral shades like caramel can be accessorized with any shade from cream to bronze to bright pinks and blues.

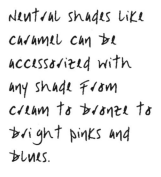

slinky minx

Jersey doesn't have to be casual! It's super-slinky which means your dress will hang beautifully from the slimmest part of your gorgeous bod. The on-trend tie front has a dual purpose – you can fit the dress perfectly to your waist, and the tie itself will conceal your yummy tummy. Bold bling, like these chunky bangles and necklace, work perfectly against this simple base.

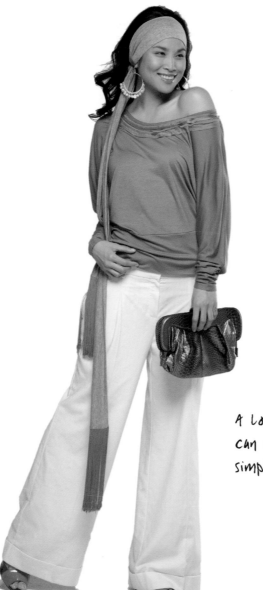

Gok's sneaky style tip
Hoop earrings always add a touch of boho cool to your outfit.

A long jersey scarf can add drama to a simple ensemble.

Off-the-shoulder Seduction

Guess what, saucy? The sexiest looks aren't always about skin-tight shapes and flashing that flesh. You'll look fabulously sensual in this loose drapey top and wide trousers. A glimpse of that gorgeous shoulder and that elegant collarbone will always be seductive, at any age, and is very slimming! Slinky jersey skims without being clingy, so it's a perfect fabric to drape across those beautiful curves.

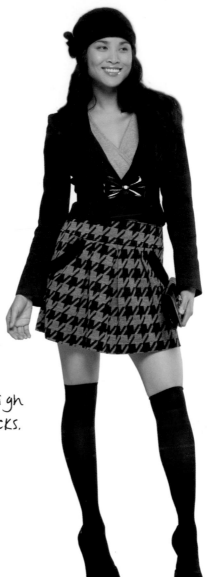

if you're too thigh
shy for long socks,
try foxy black
opaque tights.

Pretty Preppy

This is your super-cute preppy look, my angel! A flippy jersey skirt is a fun style statement, especially in a bold print like this one! Keep your top half fitted and sleek; a simple wrap-top layers neatly under a tight-cropped jacket. And an eye-catching belt keeps the focus on your amazing teeny waist. Keeping your outfit to one tone adds sophistication to your overall look.

Sometimes less is more. A beautiful coloured top doesn't need to be crowded with accessories.

Buy simple shapes in bold clear colours like this.

Bold And Bright

Sometimes the simplest ideas are the best, eh honey? Basics can look brilliant in bold colours. This bright sexy blue top is so simple, but the combination of colour, flattering style and minute detail in the twisted straps make this a wow piece. All you need are some classic, neutral wide-legged trousers and low-key flip-flops to really show it off. A really cool confident look!

Add a leather belt to cinch it round your foxy waist.

Three-quarter sleeves are great for styling; let a coloured jumper or long gloves peek out.

Big Entrance Elegance

Now that's what I call an arrival, lady! You can still make a big style statement in outerwear. You will really get noticed en route with a coat that is as flamboyant as a dress. Look for a coat with stylish detailing like the pussy bow necktie and wide sleeves here. Add a brooch to keep the look retro and on-trend.

These chunky necklaces keep the emphasis on the cool drapey Tee, not the plain polo neck base.

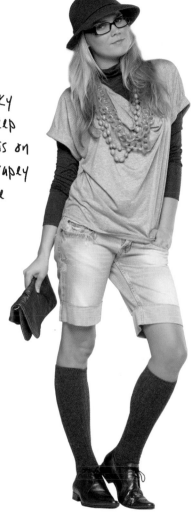

You can wear your favourite summer dress all year round by adding layers underneath!

Doubly Cool

You will look so cool in this street-style outfit; the short-sleeved baggy tee looks sassy worn over a polo neck, and your arms will look super-slim! Layer cut-off shorts with thick tights or knee-high socks when the weather's not as hot as you are.

Sexy Seventies

Cardigans aren't the only way to layer on a cold day! Keep the focus on your foxy silhouette by wearing a sassy dress over a fitted polo neck. This is your sexy Seventies look — with knee-high boots and a long necklace over the polo neck!

Gok's sneaky style tip
open-toed shoes don't
need to be saved for
summer — they look
foxy worn with opaque
tights or long socks.

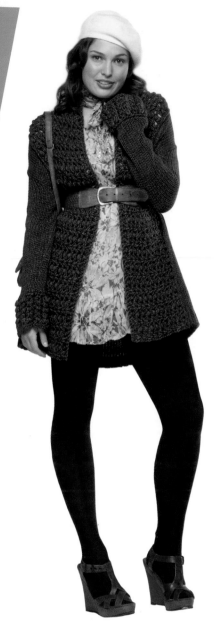

it's easier to cinch in
the waist of a cardigan
with a leather belt
than a knitted one, and a
contrasting colour will
focus eyes on your waist.

Cardi-coat Queen

A big chunky knit is a great alternative to a coat, because it becomes part of your outfit rather than just covering it up! You can still show off your dress by belting a 'cardi-coat' open, and revealing just a column of what's underneath makes your silhouette appear super-slim. All eyes will be on you, my foxy lady!

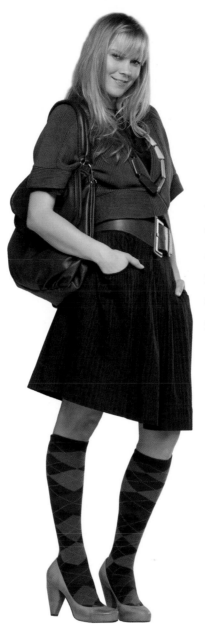

For those days when you're in between a coat and a jacket, a loose, short-sleeved cardigan makes a fashion-savvy solution.

Fit Bird

You can pile on those layers without adding bulk to your beautiful booty! With an outfit like this, you can still keep all eyes on your weeny waist. A cardigan jacket with a fitted hem, a wide skirt with a figure-hugging waistband and a bold, cinching belt all show off that awesome hourglass you got going on!

Jackets & Coats

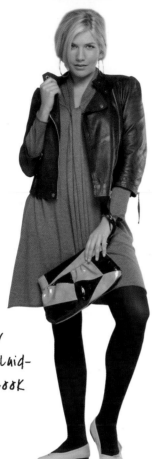

Add foxy confidence to a trench coat by turning up that collar.

Three-quarter sleeves add a laid-back casual look to a leather jacket.

Biker Babe

The leather biker jacket is another modern design classic you'll have in your wardrobe for years. But you don't always have to wear it with denim. It can also give a tough urban edge to your sexy Saturday-night dress, without covering it up. Wear with bright flats for a super-sexy finish.

All-weather Chic

Is there anything sexier than a curvy woman in a classic trench coat? This coat will keep you looking cool whatever the weather throws at you. Belt it across your slimmest part to keep you looking super-toned in all weathers, or keep it open and cinched at the back to reveal what's underneath.

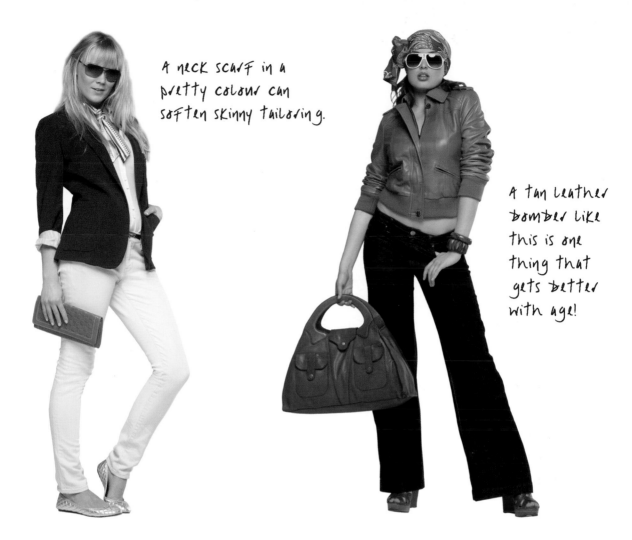

A neck scarf in a pretty colour can soften skinny tailoring.

A tan leather bomber like this is one thing that gets better with age!

Eurotrash Jacket

Honey, it's time to join the jet set! A smart blazer will instantly give slim jeans and simple flat pumps a 'grown-up' European look. A blazer cut shorter and narrower than a suit jacket is the perfect light cover-up for the summer, and looks fabulously sexy. Roll up those sleeves for an even more confident look.

Disco Cool

High-waisted flares are your chance to be one of Charlie's Angels! Worn with stacked platform heels your legs will look like they go on for ever! A cropped jacket will show off that higher waist and get the full length of those lovely leggy limbs! Don't be afraid to go all-out retro by adding timeless classics.

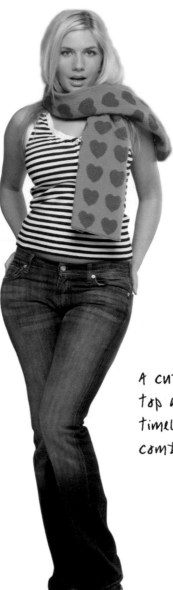

A cute stripey vest top and jeans is a timelessly classic combination.

Sassy Stripes

The all-time classic, boot-cut jean is every girl's best friend. This is a wear-with-anything jean for those days when you just want a simple classic style. A cut like this works best in darker denim, and a little faded wear on the thighs will draw the eye in and make those pins seem super-skinny.

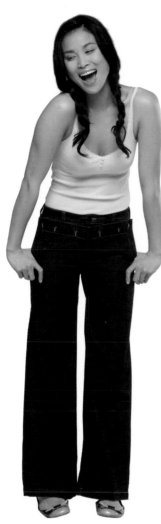

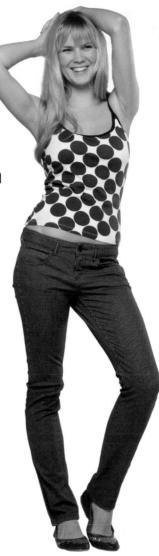

Pinstripe skinnies will elongate and slim your legs even more!

Wide-legged jeans also look casual cool with little pumps.

Navy Lady

Wide-legged sailor pants look so stylish right now! Cut straight down from your widest point to the floor, these are super-flattering with heels or flats. Make sure the waistband is just tight enough, so that the back is snug around that gorgeous bum of yours.

Skinny jeans

The vest and skinny jeans combo is your ultimate rock-chick look. Wear with flat footwear like ballet pumps for a casual, sexy finish. Jeans like these have elastic in with the denim so they hug those hips and never get saggy. A crazy, retro pattern top will distract from any midriff issues!

Accessories

Accessories are a great way to alter the look of your wardrobe staples in a matter of moments. In fact, add a basics outfit to the accessories shown here and you've got a capsule wardrobe in itself!

1 A great belt is essential for layering, adding definition, and keeping that silhouette tight and trim.

2 A simple ensemble will let oversized jewellery shine.

3 A classic riding boot will keep your feet happy (and stylish) for years. Look for a pair that really fits and flatters your legs.

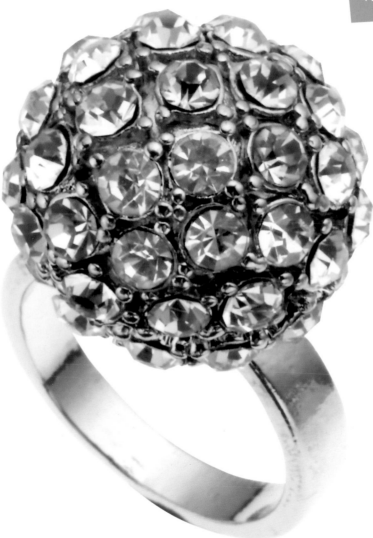

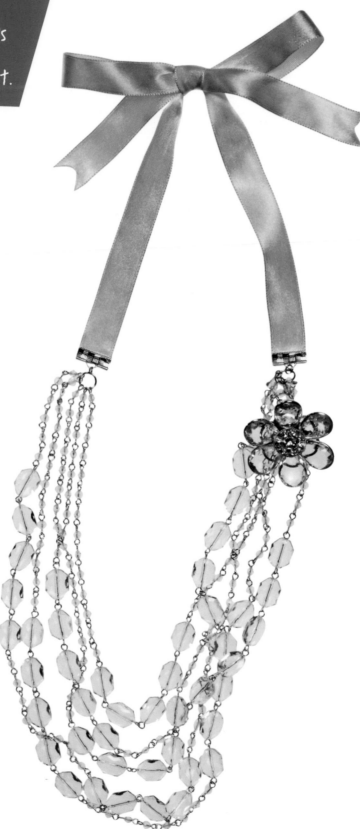

4 Long scarves aren't just for winter! Wrap one around your neck to add an extra shot of summer colour.

5 Bright accessories and shoes add an edgy pop of colour to classic neutrals like black and grey.

6 A long necklace will soften the contrast of two layered tops.

7 Let jazzy knee-high socks peek out of the top of classic tall boots.

So let's get back to basics! Short of keeping me in the back of your wardrobe, nothing's going to be more useful in helping you get a fabulous look together each morning than a selection of brilliant basics.

These basics are your New Best Friends, ready to guide you through season to season and from event to event. A set of wardrobe staples at your fingertips will make you feel like a super-confident dresser, always with something up your sleeve for whatever comes next.

These pieces are going to be the perfect way for you to wear that fabulous new top or skirt without having to wrestle with a whole new outfit. They'll each give the edgier pieces in your wardrobe an extended life just by sitting next to them. In the future, when you buy a funky new piece, you'll already have the perfect basic to go with it (which means that everything you buy will be ready-to-wear!).

There's nothing like a collection of simple pieces in your wardrobe when you're having a busy day or just want to play it chic. Once you've got them sorted, the world of style is yours for the taking!

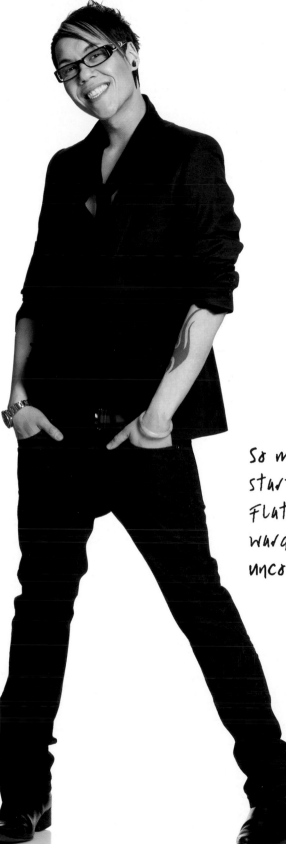

So my gorgeous, let's
start building you a
flattering and fabulous
wardrobe of simple,
uncomplicated pieces.

UNDER WEAR

Figure-fixing, flirting and femininity

- Panelling creates the illusion of a super-slim silhouette
- if you're tummy-shy wear a babydoll slip
- magic underwear with sex appeal

Honey, this is your Bond girl moment. And your 007 secret weapon in the style stakes? Underwear.

The right underwear can totally transform your booty. A smoothing and slimming pair of Gok's favourite magic pants will make you look like you've had liposuction, and a well-fitting new bra will get results as good as any boob job.

It's so worth taking the time to find your perfect set of underwear because once you've got that right, like a great haircut or finding the right foundation, everything else seems to fall into place. Of course, as well as the way your underwear can make you look (i.e. fabulously curvy), a gorgeous set of lingerie will also make you feel sexier and more feminine. Mee-ow!

Lady, you could be wearing just a simple white T-shirt and jeans, but with a foxy little lacy bra and knicker set underneath you'll have an über-confident glow all day that everyone will notice (but nobody will be able to work out). Unless, of course, you want them to …

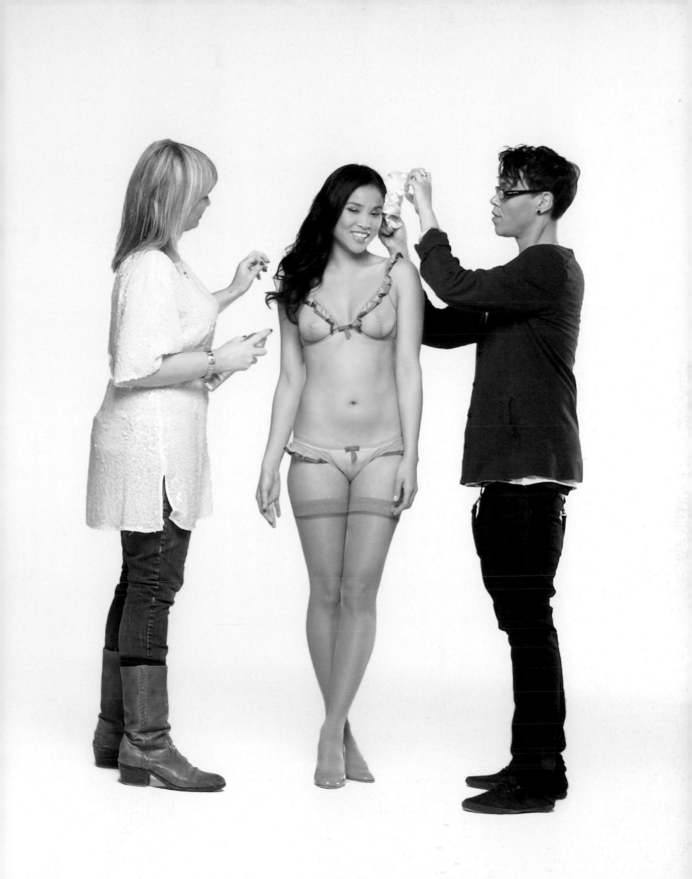

COLOUR & PATTERN

Colourful patterns and prints are super-cute for the day. Maybe there's a strict dress code in your office, but that doesn't mean you can't wear bright pink stripy underwear (just be careful it doesn't show through when you're wearing a white cotton shirt).

Off duty, if you've got fabulously coloured underwear why hide it? Have a cheeky coloured strap peeking out from a vest top, or at the shoulders of a slash-neck Tee. Or let your crisp white shirt reveal just a sneaky glimpse of pretty lace bra.

Pale pink and nude shades will make you look chic and sensual without being too OTT. These will work best under your white shirts and T-shirts (beware: white under white always shows through). Lacy fabrics or funky prints like polka dots add a kick to quieter colours – he won't know what's hit him!

And how to stop the classic black-and-red combo looking too tarty (although let's not forget, tarty can be fun too)? Wear simple, streamlined shapes for an über-classy after-dark look.

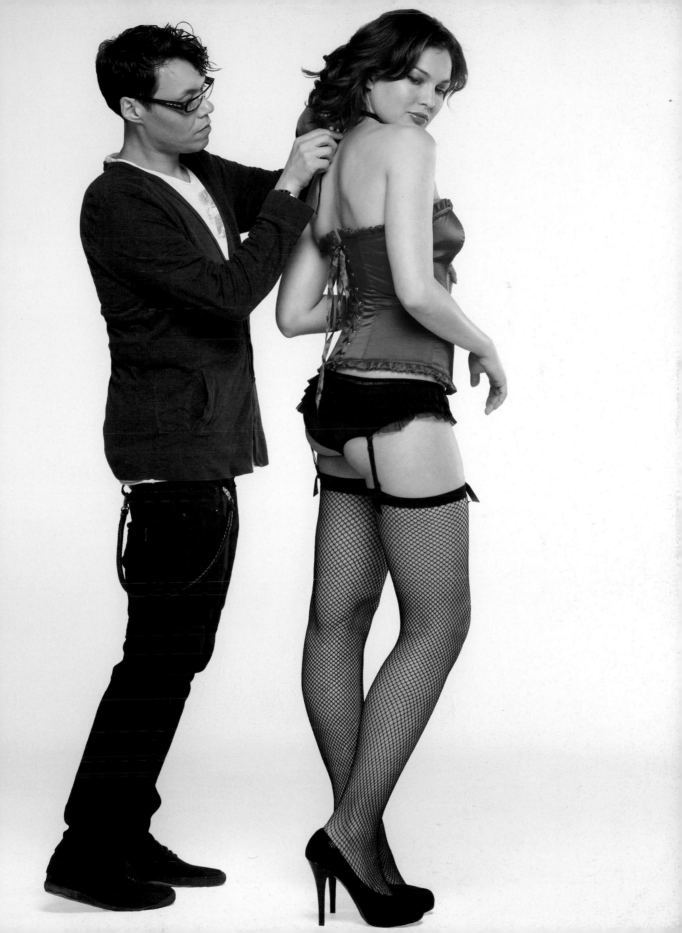

MIX & MATCH

Mismatched underwear was once a big no-no. Your mother always warned you not to mismatch your underwear in case you got hit by a bus. Well, sorry Mum, but mix and match is now a cool look, and when your fella sees you, it's him who's going to feel like he's been hit by a bus!

The reason mixing it up can be so hot? It's great for figure fixing. If you're boobalicious you can wear your favourite plain structured bra with some hip-boosting vertical stripe briefs. Pretty pears can keep their pretty pair in a bold print push-up bra, and you can then pick out one of the darker colours in the print for a hip-diminishing high leg brief.

The trick with mixing is to take one colour through the whole set, to make the mix look deliberate rather than accidental. So a pale blue bra can work with cute stripy knickers, if there's a matching blue in the stripes. Easy! Have a look at my mixed up combo in this chapter to see it in action.

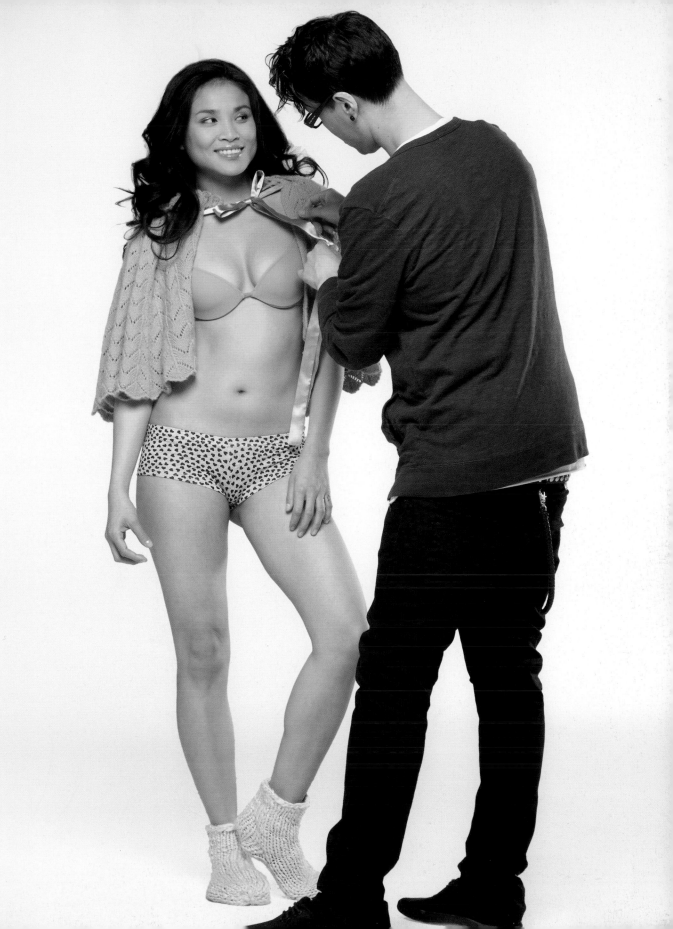

BEAUTY

Of course, there's nothing more seductive than sexy lingerie, but don't stop there. Think about the whole ensemble rather than just the lingerie itself. There's probably going to be a lot of that gorgeous skin on show, so remember to moisturize, crack open the bronzer and use a shimmering powder where the light hits your skin. Smokin'.

Keeping hair messy and tousled will give an 'undone' twist to even the most boned of bedroom outfits.

Nude, natural make-up will accentuate that going-to-bed vibe, so work those subtle tones and keep it simple. A little lip gloss and a swipe of liquid eyeliner will work wonders for your seductive prowess, and add some blusher on the apples of your cheeks for an instant 'so pleased to see you' flush ... and don't forget to dust between those sexy bangers for the illusion of an even deeper cleavage.

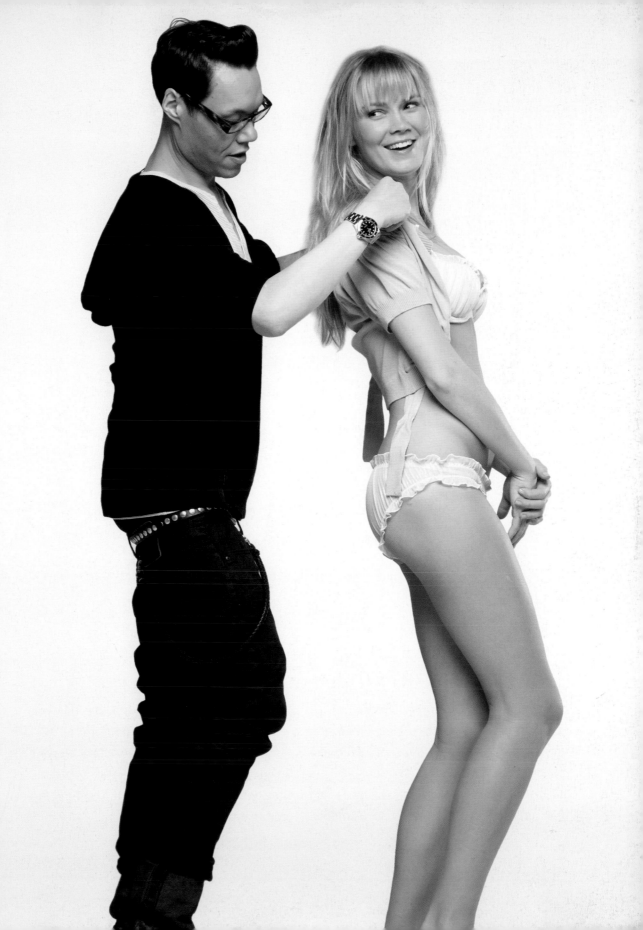

Magic Underwear

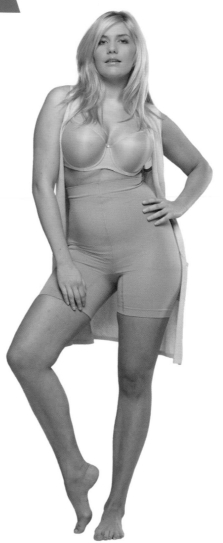

Why just save your magic underwear for going out? Now you can look a million dollars in your jeans and T-shirt too!

Smooth operator

First things first. Let's bring out the best of your curves by smoothing that silhouette. So, abracadabra: magic pants, to make that scrummy tummy and juicy thighs practically disappear (don't worry — it's just an illusion). A fabulous silky-smooth seamless, invisible-toned bra like this will give the impression of nothing more than a perfect rack underneath your elegant evening number. In fact it is all so seam-free, you'll have him thinking you're going commando (you tease).

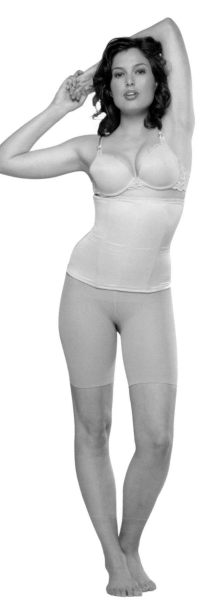

A waist-cinching tummy panel like this is the modern-day corset – but feel free to play the helpless heroine.

Wonder Woman

Think of this underwear 'outfit' as your secret superhero-wear: pushing everything up, up and way-hey! Honey, nothing is escaping from this ensemble! A secret tummy flattener like this will smooth your beautiful belly and help accentuate your waspish waist. Add a pair of thigh-smoothing shorts and boost those beautiful bangers with a boosting bra, and you'll get 10/10 for the perfect figure of 8. Your secret superpower? Being able to slay men with a single wiggle.

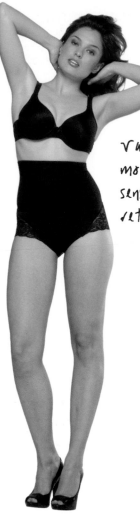

vamp up that movie star sensuality with retro-sexy heels!

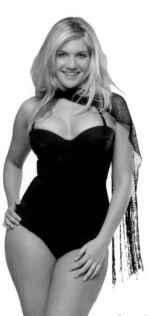

An all-in-one like this can be just as hot as a matching set!

Screen Siren Sexy

Yes, magic underwear can be as gorgeous as you are! Think Fifties screen siren in this vampy black two-piece. Decadent detailing like this luxurious lace will keep you looking elegantly erotic. Best of all, foxy-but-firm pants will smooth and boost your sexy tum and bum. And a slinky padded satin bra will boost those beautiful boobs.

Drama Queen

This, my gorgeous, is your ultimate Little Black Dress (the smallest one you'll ever wear!). And like your favourite LBD this foxy number is slimming, sexy and oh-so-sophisticated. The all-in-one shape keeps everything tight-to-the-torso (we're talking awesome hourglass), and the low-cut, built-in bra will give you a décolletage to die for.

Sheer panelling in a darker colour lets you play peekaboo, revealing just a hint of thong.

A frilly hem will draw attention to the tops of saucy stockings. Scorching!

Moulin rouge

Just like you, a flirty outfit like this has it all going on! A burlesque-style babydoll with a cheeky top hat and stockings is a great way to put on a spectacular show!

And the best ticket in the house is the balconette – the contrasting detailing around the cups will ensure your bangers are the main attraction. Encore!

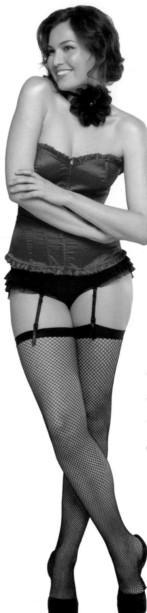

Gok's sneaky style tip
A more modern way to wear red and black: simple streamlined shapes look ultra sophisticated.

The boning in a bustier will keep your fabulous body looking perfect until you want to reveal all.

Ooh La La!

Suddenly your bedroom is a boudoir! A boned bustier like this is pure, unadulterated naughtiness (especially in saucy scarlet), and frilly knickers can give a touch of Parisian cancan glamour. Those classic touches, like fishnet stockings, suspender belts and high heels, will never fail. Ooh la la …

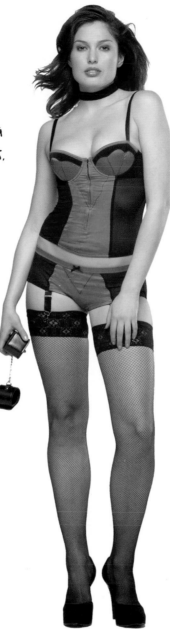

A choker necklace adds a subtle touch of sexiness, and focuses attention on those perky bangers – just use ribbon.

Gok's sneaky style tip
And why not go all the way – with some saucy cuffs!

Basque Babe

Who says saucy underwear can't flatter your fabulous figure? Panelling like this in a contrasting colour draws the eye in and creates the illusion of a super-slim silhouette, all the way down your gorgeous bod. Wider brief-style pants will flatter curvaceous hips. Saucy stockings will drive your fella wild!

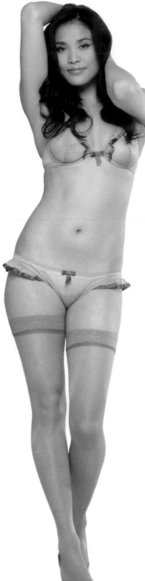

Ruffle hem knickers will make your hips and thighs look even slimmer! Yum!

Au Natural naughtiness

What could be more seductive than ... nude? Okay, beige might not seem like your most inspiring choice, but you're going to look über-sophisticated in this subtly sexy colour. Some minxy detailing like the contrasting bows and ruffles will add flirty femininity. Best of all, you'll look even more naked than you are! Naughty!

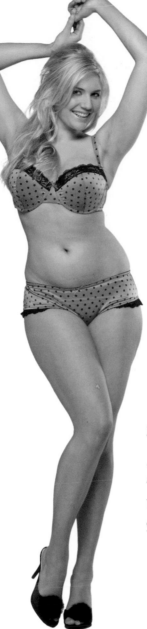

Bright colours look great against tanned and darker skin tones; wear this for some summer lovin'.

Summer lovin'

Give him an eyeful ... of bright sexy colour in the bedroom! A bold colour like this shows confidence and style and you naughty lady have both. The lace trim along the bra and knickers keeps it sexy as well as cute. And the cheeky polka-dot pattern is totally on-trend right now. Wowsers!

A little ribbon
detailing on the bra
will add a delicate
touch of femininity.
Gorgeous!

Rainbow babe

Well, good morning! Colourful printed lingerie is a great addition to your underwear drawer! I guarantee it'll put a smile on your face (and his!) first thing.

Stripes are a fun fresh look for the summer. And don't be afraid of horizontal stripes; they'll accentuate your curves and give you a weeny waist.

Sometimes, my gorgeous, keeping things hidden is even more sexy than putting them on show.

Mix super-bright colours like these with barely-there natural tights.

Sixties sex kitten

Well, bonjour Brigitte Bardot! You will look like a Sixties sex-kitten in this cute babydoll slip. A flirty shape like this can give you a little extra coverage for when you're feeling body shy (or like a bit of a tease!), and a colourful pattern will refocus attention on those luscious limbs and lady-lumps. Now start practising that pout ...

Breakfast in Bed

A slinky knitted cardigan flatters your silhouette better than a thick towelling robe.

Don't be afraid to mix prints in similar colours for a casual mix and match vibe.

Cosy Cutie

How cute are you, my gorgeous? A cotton floral number like this is perfect for weekend lounging (and lovin'). A delicate floral pattern will make you look feminine and pretty, and a soft cardigan knit makes a chic dressed-up dressing gown.

Separates are a great solution
option for my boobalicious
babes! update your favourite
bra with cute new knickers.

Minxy Mismatch

This, my gorgeous, is Gok's tutorial in mixing and matching and still looking stylish. Choose one colour – like this pretty ballet pink – and take it through the whole outfit for a cute, sexy look. He won't be able to keep his hands off you!

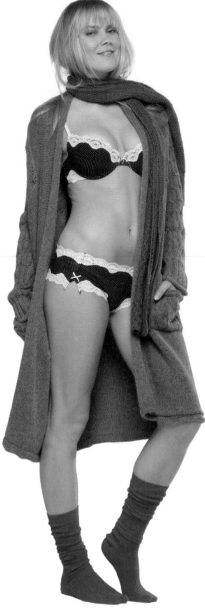

Contrasting detailing
Like the lace here
draws all attention to
your beautiful boobs.

BLACK To Bed

Now, repeat after Gok, 'I can't go wrong in monochrome!' Black and white is the fastest way for you to look classic and coordinated with a minimum of effort. French cami-knickers like these are super- comfy and very classy, and a simple underwired bra like this will keep your fabulous chest in the right place all day (and night) long. A cardi-dressing gown and cute slouch socks give you a dressed undress-me look. Naughty!

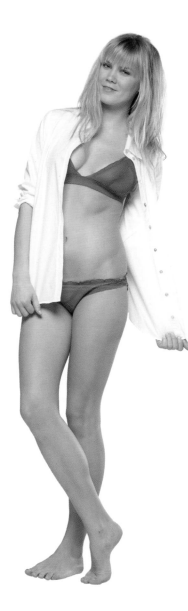

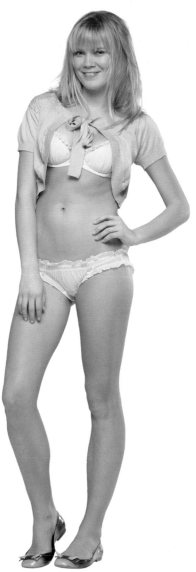

Simple cream and nude sets are less visible under white or sheer fabrics than bright white sets!

Sheer Sex

Let's keep your complexion sexy in a simple but sizzling set. Mid-tones like turquoise, purple or coral look fabulously flattering with all skin tones. A sheer mesh bra is ideal for dressed-down daywear. And non-wired bra styles are perfect for you, my small chested chica!

Cream Dream

The simplest ideas are often the best. Pale colours look soft and feminine, and a little lace detail at the top of the bra and on the edge of the knickers adds a little pretty-pretty for my girly girl. With an outfit this playful he'll be hoping for more than just breakfast in bed.

Accessories

Chilling out doesn't have to mean slobbing out!
For easy-like-Sunday-morning dressing it's all about
feeling comfy and looking chic – just add some
fabulous accessories! And while bedroom dressing is
really about less is more, you can style up your look
with some of the sexy suggestions here.

1   A shrug or knitted capelet is a cute
    alternative to a dressing gown – cosy
    without covering you up!

2   Colourful slouchy socks are the new
    slippers; so soft he won't be able to
    resist snuggling up!

3   Hold-ups are just as foxy as suspenders
    but a whole lot comfier – sex on legs!

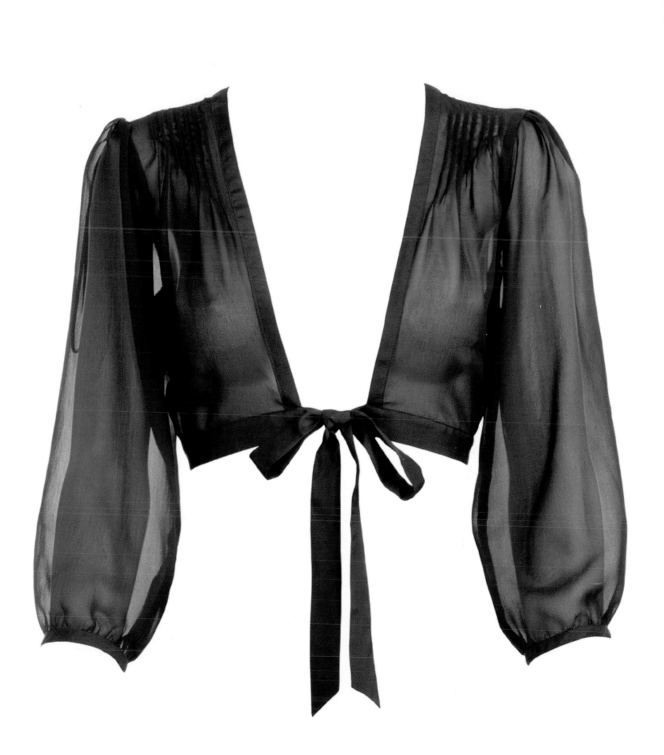

4 Heels add height and shape to those pins; über-bare backless mules are the most flattering of all.

5 For a sexy burlesque show with an audience of one, try a totally Moulin Rouge tiny top hat or saucy long gloves. Encore!

6 High socks aren't just cosy; they're cheerleader-sexy too.

7 A mesh scarf adds some flirty glamour to your look, you total vamp!

Gok's sneaky style tip

Peep-toed high-heeled shoes are retro-flirty and will elongate your gorgeous pins (don't forget that pedicure!).

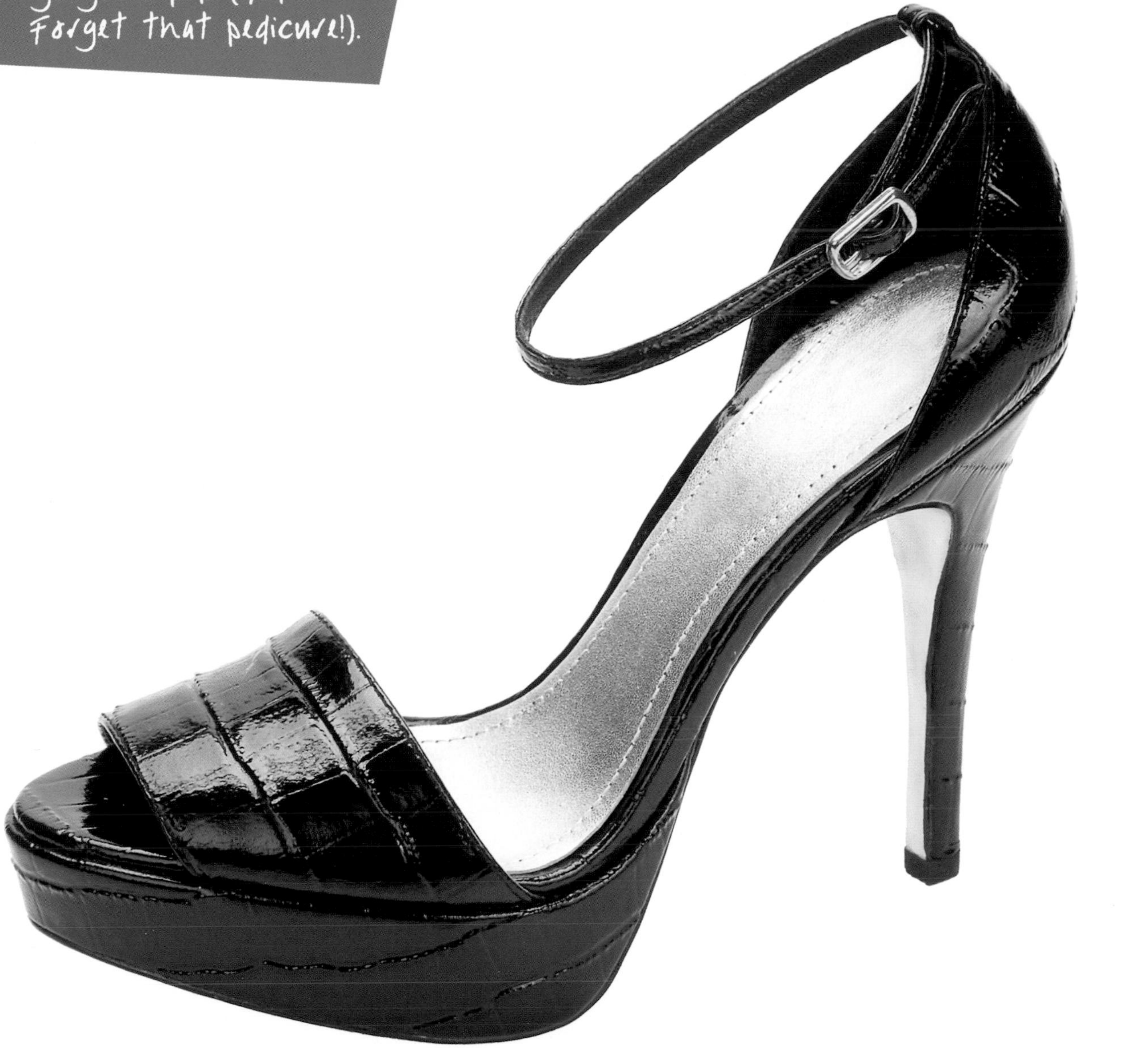

Gorgeous, when it comes to underwear I am not taking any excuses! Your perfect underwear will trim, tone and smooth that fabulous body of yours, leaving nothing sagging or bagging and without a stitch of surgery.

Whatever you're wearing, and no matter what occasion, wearing the right underwear can dramatically alter the way the rest of your outfit looks. Don't think that because it's underneath your clothes it doesn't make a difference! Good underwear is like magic dust, transforming a good outfit into one that's great.

For those occasions where underwear is all you're going to wear, you can look foxy and fabulous by wearing the best underwear for your shape and by really taking care of that super-soft skin.

So my gorgeous, whether it's for the bedroom or the boardroom, for a weekend wedding or a weekend in bed, it's time to chuck out those old bras and head to the lingerie department. Girlfriend, we're going shopping!

Apart from making you look totally drop-dead gorgeous, underwear can be the sexiest thing on the planet.

WORK WEAR

Professional, polished and pulled-together

- how to stay cool when it's hot in the city
- office to out-on-the-town outfits
- catwalk cool that stands out from the suits

I'm sure you've seen the movie *Working Girl*. It's one of my favourite movies ever; those huge big-shouldered suits are a fashion moment in time I will never get tired of watching!

Happily for you, office elegance has loosened up somewhat since the Eighties, and these days the look is more about stylish polish than power dressing.

Chic tailored trousers and sexy figure-flattering dresses are your new 'suits'. Your working wardrobe might even just be a smarter version of the clothes you like to wear anyway, and dress-down Friday might mean pulling out some of your weekend-wear a day early.

DRESSES

You know why dresses work for work? Because, like you, they're über-efficient; they look beautifully pulled together, and in zero time.

Crisp, tailored shapes work best: sleeveless shifts and shirt dresses. And let's not forget the wear-anywhere sophistication of the classic wrap dress.

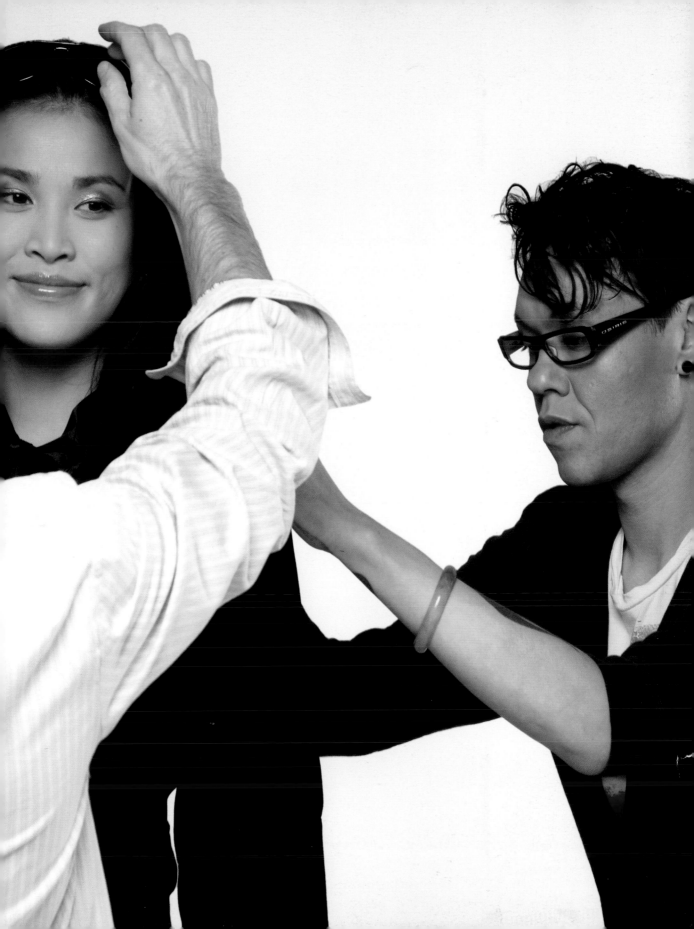

SUITS

Suits you madam! A classic men's three-piece trouser suit is a seriously foxy look for the office. Show them who wears the trousers with the full Annie Hall look – sexy Savile Row-style, with a sleek polo neck sweater. Better yet, get suited and booted with some leg-lengthening high-heeled ankle boots.

A modern minimalist look will keep you looking sleek and chic. Discreet details like flat-fronted slim-leg trousers or a single-breasted jacket with narrow lapels will always impress. Or go Chicago City slicker. Wear just a waistcoat with a white shirt and wide trousers – a curve-loving but formal look for corporate cool. And watch out for pinstripe fabrics which are businesslike and elongate your body.

Your perfect skirt suit will be serious but feminine, for a touch of retro-sexy style. Even the smartest tailored suits can have subtle sensual details to keep you feeling womanly; a gentle puff sleeve on a jacket, rounded pockets or lapels, a flared sleeve or hem. And a tightly tailored waist on a jacket is a winner every time; add a contrasting belt to keep the focus on your hourglass shape.

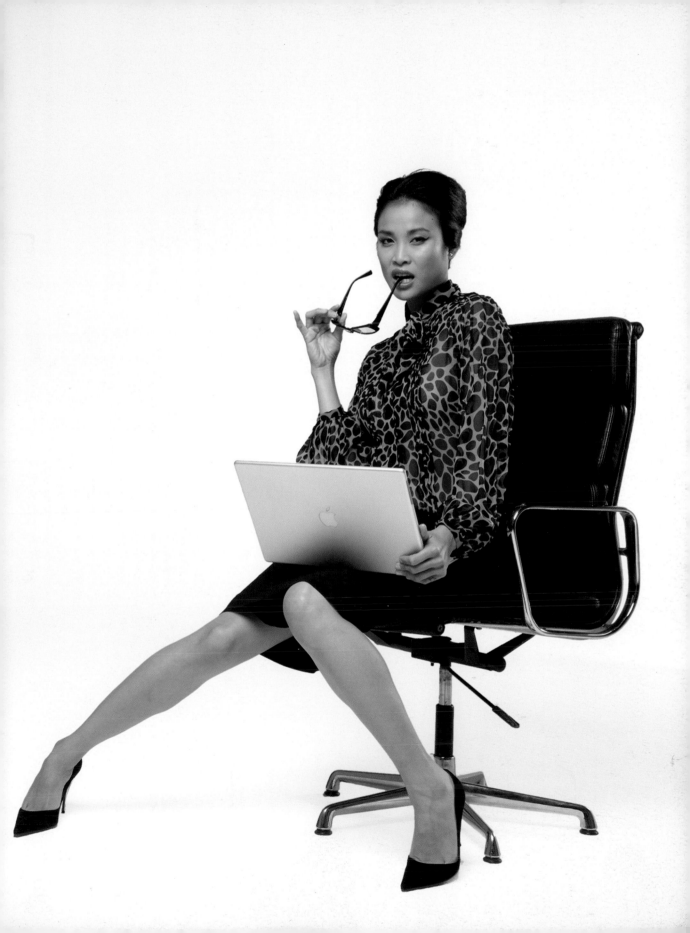

OVERTIME

Sometimes your office outfits will need to do over-time; yes, I'm talking about client entertaining. But honey, it's easy to find outfits to take you from desk to drinks party, and here are some tips.

- Try suit shapes in evening fabrics. A smart skirt with a hint of a sheeny fabric, a tailored suit with a metallic thread running through it, or wide-legged trousers in vampy velvet will all switch from meeting room to posh restaurant.

- Blouses will keep you looking serious for day and sophisticated at night. A frilly blouse with a pencil skirt, or a bold printed or pussy-bow blouse with wide-legged trousers are perfect for the 9 to 5 and then the 5 to 9!

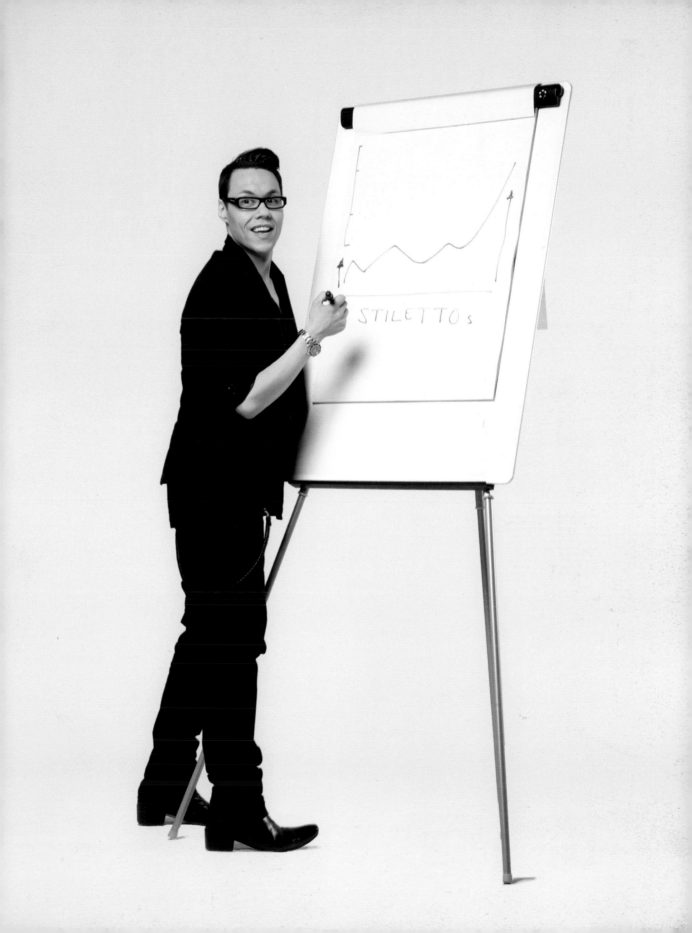

DRESS-DOWN FRIDAY

Nobody ever got fired for getting dress-down Friday wrong. But still, it's ironic that a dress code that's supposed to make you feel more relaxed at work can create the most anxiety! Bold colours are a fun way to give your seriously smart work look the day off. Swap greys, blacks and neutral shades for stronger colours like red or green.

Relax Your Fabrics

Tailoring still works for DDF, but softer fabrics will make your look seem more laid-back. A blazer-shape jacket in a fluid jersey, a neat polo shirt instead of a crisp cotton button-down, or a pencil skirt in a smart dark denim, makes a concession to casual without compromising any of your polished style.

Relax Your Shapes

A pair of wide-legged trousers, like the classic navy trousers (hello, sailor!), will feel comfy while still looking über-stylish (think Katharine Hepburn's fabulous Forties sophistication). Wear with flat shoes for the ultimate in easy chic.

The key to getting it right on dress-down Friday? Just relax, honey!

Black tights can work with a bright colour! But be sure to balance all that black with a matching necklace or belt.

The 24-hour shift

Honey, this is your summer equivalent of the wrap dress; the any time, any place, any wear sleeveless shift will keep you looking sleek, modern and über-professional in any scenario. You'll also look smokin' hot! A matching belt and bag is the ultimate chic.

With beige as your base, you can add different colours for a variety of looks – super-efficient fashion!

Super Safari

It's hot in the city! Okay, not as hot as in the jungle (although sometimes when the air-conditioning's broken …) but you get the idea. Safari is a classic style to wear in the summer. You'll look crisp and smart when the heat is on. A traditional shirt dress looks sharp without being too buttoned-up.

wear it another way:
a short-sleeve crew
neck would be a
chic cooler weather
alternative (think
fifties sweater girl).

Retro sexy

Work it, girlfriend! Just because you're at work, doesn't mean you can't show off that awesome silhouette! This retro sexy look is smart enough to take you into any boardroom. A pencil skirt with a kick hem looks formal and foxy, and a light pretty blouse balances the tailoring with a softer femininity.

This is trendy enough for you to go straight to a club from the boardroom; and why not add a funky hat on the way?

A waistcoat can be your smart alternative to a jacket when the temperature rises, Hot stuff.

City Slicker

Check you, slinky city slicker! It might be a man's world (or at least, let them think that sometimes) but your take on the traditional three-piece suit will show them who's boss.

Wide trousers like these are fashionable and flattering. The tailored waistcoat will really emphasize that waist, and is saucily low-cut without being revealing.

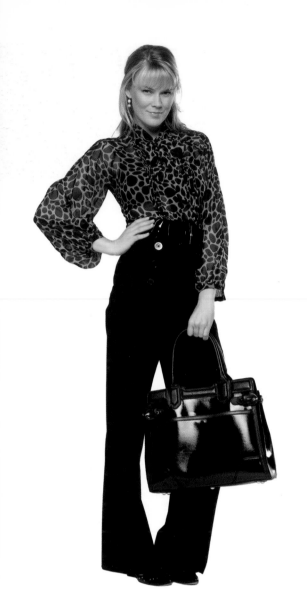

This will be your number one office staple for taking you from 9 to 5 and beyond.

Boardroom Bold

Nothing's more professional than confidence, which is why bold prints can really work for you in the office. A sheer fabric or a bow neck will soften the look and add femininity, against some on-trend trousers. Keep your trousers simply tailored and chic.

All Wrapped Up

Like you, the wrap dress is great at doing overtime. The super-flattering frock was originally designed for confident career women of the Seventies, and honey, there ain't nothin' else like it! Formal enough for meetings yet comfy enough to wear all day, it's also super-sexy.

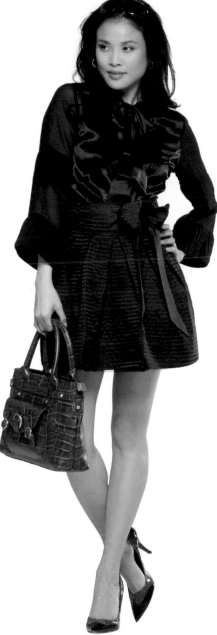

Gok's sneaky style tip
Bell-shaped skirts like this are perfect for you, my gorgeous broad!

wear it another way: black opaque tights and ballet pumps would also look fabulous with this skirt.

Blouse Babe

This is your sexy executive look, lady. Dressy takes on the classic blouse-and-skirt combo, which will keep you looking corporate-smart at work, then cocktail-chic for entertaining clients. Shiny fabrics look polished for day, but luxurious for evening.

Own your suit, Lady! Rolling up jacket sleeves is a stylishly relaxed look (and shows you mean business).

Don't forget your favourite leg-lengthening trick of matching your trousers and your shoes, even for grey!

Grey Fox

Suits you! A slim-cut trouser suit makes a simple but chic style statement for work. Discreet details like thin lapels, flat-fronted slim trousers and a subtle colour like grey all add to its modern minimalism, instantly making you look quietly confident (promotion, anyone?). A kick of colour underneath will show you're bright as well as quietly efficient. Heels are a must, adding height and authority to your look.

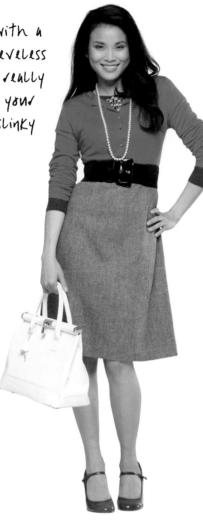

Starting with a fitted sleeveless dress will really streamline your look, you slinky minx.

Vertical pinstripes are professional and slimming, foxy!

Prim And Super-slim

Air-con, stuffy offices, naughtiness in the stationery cupboard (ahem) — layering is your only way to survive modern workplaces. Here, we've piled on a dress, a long-sleeved sweater and a cardigan, without piling on the pounds! Just make sure to layer fitted shapes, and super-fine knits, and use a belt to define the waist and pull the layers together.

Pinafore Princess

Suits you, madam! A suit and tie doesn't have to mean trousers, working girl. This foxy dress and jacket combo is a workwear capsule wardrobe in itself! This look is smartly professional while still giving a nod to fashion with the layering and the cheeky tie. And the dress's stream-lined silhouette will be fabulously figure-flattering.

Shorter skirts look less revealing with opaque tights underneath.

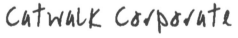

Catwalk Corporate

Every boss wants clued-up staff, which is why a contemporary cut of suit shows you're the (super)model employee. There's no need to leave your love of fashion at home, so choose a suit like this, with its ultra-cool cropped jacket and sculptural skirt. An interesting fabric, like this muted metallic material, will also help you stand out from the other suits.

Preppy Princess

This preppy-with-a-twist style will show how super-switched-on you are, my office angel. By adding a smart short-sleeved shirt to your going-out skinny trousers and sexy stilettos you can turn your look from evening to efficient. The great thing about this look: you'll always look keen, together and ready for action (however hungover you are).

Swap that starched shirt for a T-shirt!

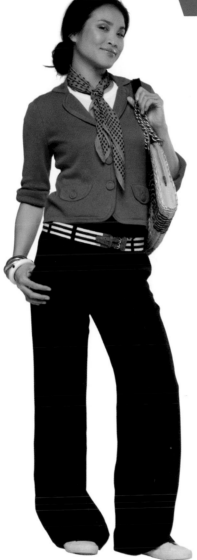

Mix and mismatch

There are other ways to relax at work than playing on Facebook, you know (I can see you!). For DDFs loosen up your work look by wearing tailored shapes in softer fabrics like this jersey jacket. Wide-legged trousers will keep you looking laidback but still professional. Mixing and matching jackets and trousers instantly makes you look less formal (and you get more from your wardrobe; sneaky!)

Accessories

Accessories can promote any outfit from business to pleasure. For those unexpected invitations for client entertaining, let your desk drawer double as a dressing-up box – keep a supply of accessories like evening tights, a clutch bag and a classic pair of stilettos there. Here are my suggestions for nifty pieces to help you really work that look!

1 Hate heels? A pair of immaculate white plimsolls will make you look casual but smart. And loafers are sophisticated and on-trend, and oh-so-comfy.

2 Simple fuss-free accessories are just the job for your clean, streamlined style.

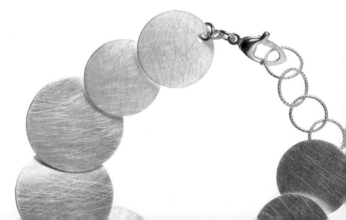

Gok's sneaky style tip

Shoe boots are seriously edgy right now, and can look just as as professional as your classic court shoes.

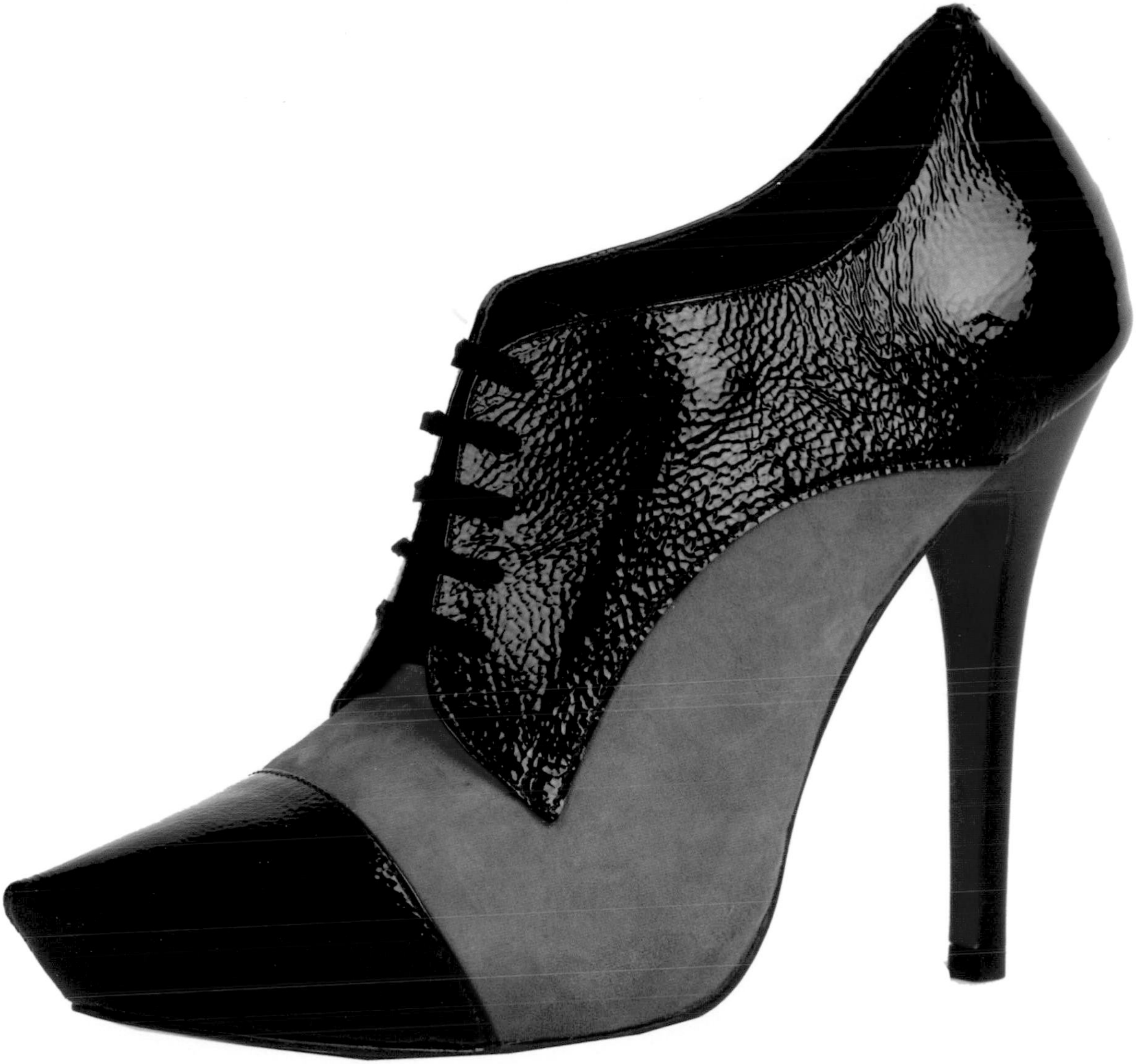

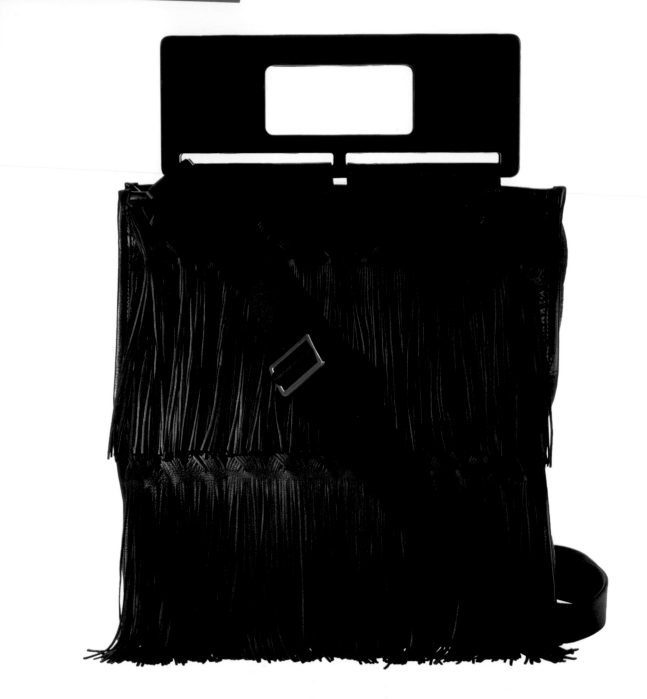

3 Plain polished accessories work perfectly against busy prints.

4 Swap your tights from sheer to fishnet to sauce your work look up for the evening!

5 A wide belt will accentuate your fabulous silhouette without being too body-conscious for the workplace.

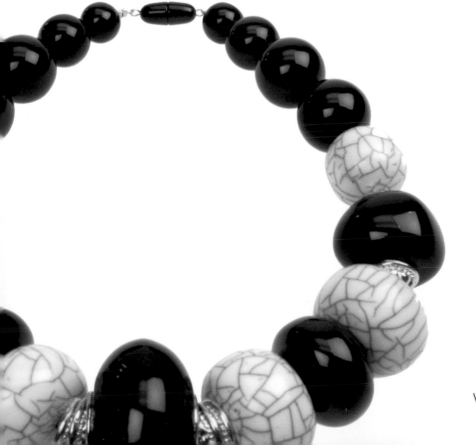

There's no need to worry about your work wardrobe. Just think about the clothes you like to wear, the ones that make you feel gorgeous, that flatter your fabulous figure and that are comfortable for you to be in all day long.

Once you've thought about those wardrobe faves then we can start to think about styling them for the office. Honey, what's the point of buying something 'just for work' if you wouldn't wear it at the weekend? You spend most of your week in your work outfits, so they need to be practical and comfortable, as well as making you feel super-confident and able to take on anything.

We've taken a sartorial step into the boardroom and gone through all those possibilities that the world of work throws up, from entertaining clients to formal meetings and dress-down Friday. My gorgeous girl, from this point forward these are your new favourite excuses to dress up and look fabulous.

So step away from the photocopier, honey, because we're going shopping. Let's show the world you mean business!

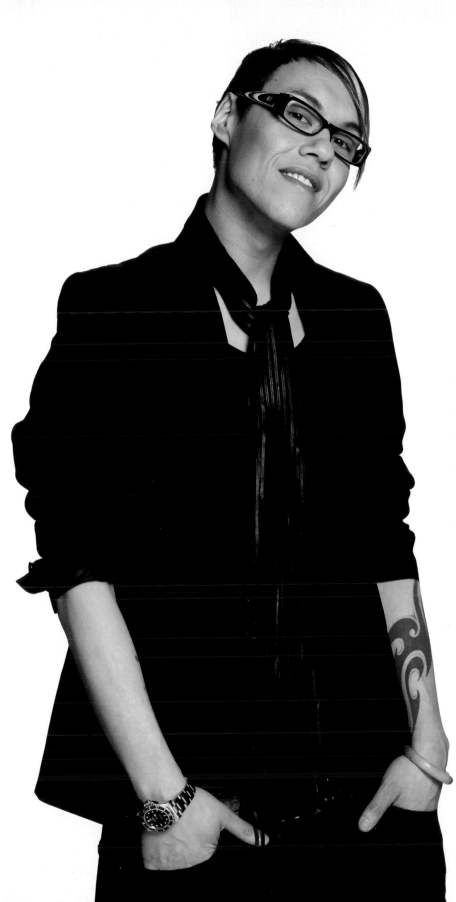

You're already a superstar so let's project that outwards and let the world see you in action, you confident diva.

GOING OUT

Funky, fun and fashionable

- easy ways to jazz up your jeans
- no-brainer, on-trend clubbing looks
- what to wear for that work do

There's nothing like a night on the town to show the world how completely fabulous you are! After all, it would be a crime to keep your beautiful self at home!

Whether you're meeting friends for a drink in the pub, going to a dinner party, dancing all night long or going to a swanky bash, going out is all about having fun. And a big part of that fun is going to be getting you all dressed up (and honey, I mean UP).

A GIRL'S BEST FRIEND

Trust me, nothing showcases your curves better than those blue beauties when you're off to paint the town red. Sitting down at the pub all evening, or dancing on the bar all night, a pair of jeans are your kick-back-and-look-cool solution. Oh, and unless you're super-tall, buy jeans that hit the floor when you're barefoot and wear them with heels to lengthen those lovely legs.

Skinnies are your edgy rock-chick option! So work the look with faded washes and fuller volume tops like baggy Tees or swing jackets. You can team with ballet flats or try tucking into tall boots. Flares will

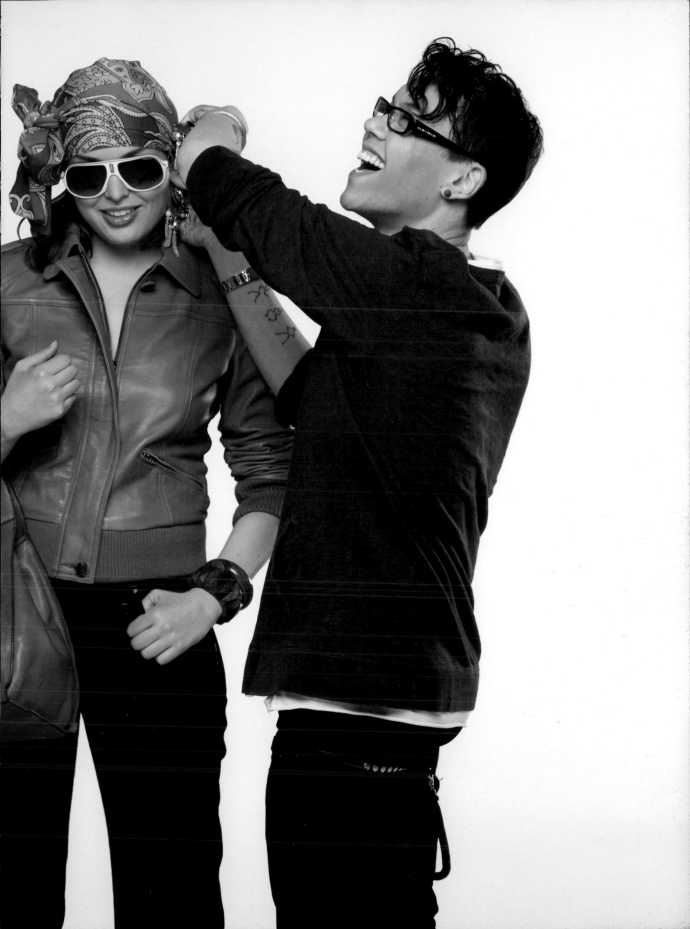

give you a touch of seventies glamour! These sexy babies look great with a feminine blouse, or simple v-neck Tees and platform heels – foxy! Fancy feeling like a Fashionista? Try a high-waisted style. These hold you in around the midriff, so tuck in a tight top, with flashing detailing like a scoop neck and three-quarter sleeves. Add a narrow belt and the highest chunky heels you can find; the more height the better! And finally the classic slim-cut jean is very classy in a dark indigo, and you'll look very polished and grown-up wearing smart pieces like a fitted jacket and loafers. Love. It!

TOP NIGHT OUT

Darling, you are a top bird! And I'm going to find you something to wear with those jeans that will bring out your 'wow' factor from your tasty waist upwards. You're going to become one of the glitterati, my sweet. A sparkly top is fashion's answer to a glass of champagne. So let's toast your bangers and get some fizz back in your wardrobe! A strappy embellished vest is your sexy option (and looser styles skim stomachs but still look slinky); you can't go wrong with a vest top and jeans for a night out!

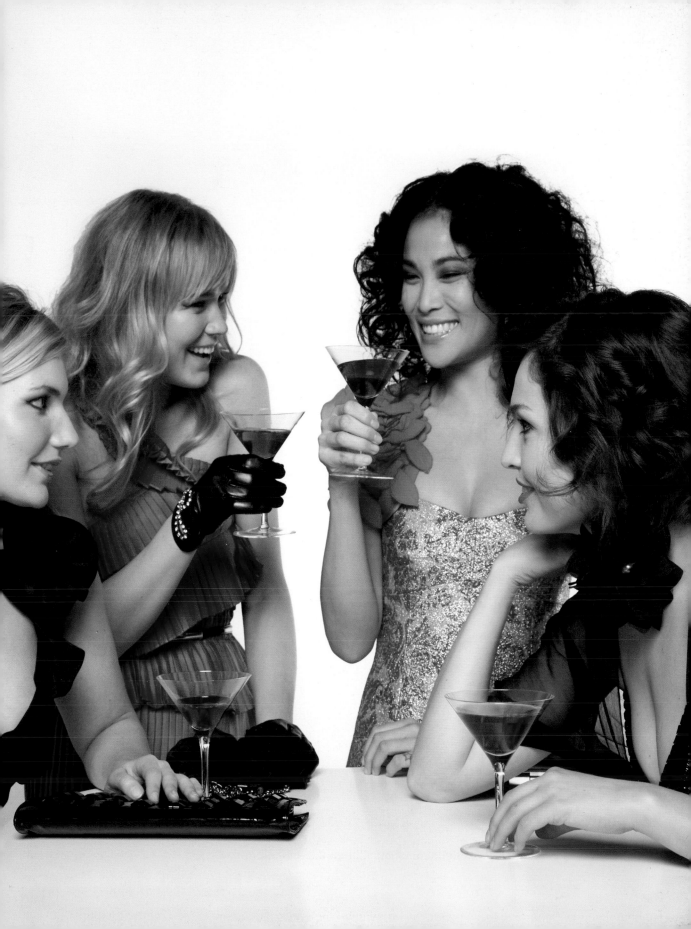

FUN FROCKS

A fun frock is going to be your jump-in-run-out speedy style solution. Dresses are so versatile for all your play dates; they can be dressed up in heels for dancing or worn to the cinema or pub with funky flat boots or ballet pumps and opaque tights.

The key to a great dress is finding something a bit different that's going to look gorgeous just on you. So what nifty detailing is going to rock your frock? Everybody loves the little black dress (it's a classic)! But finding a dress in a wow colour will really show you intend to brighten everyone's night out (as well as your own sexy complexion!). And if you really want to go for it, clashing is cool and instantly breathes new life into dresses! Stick to the same shades; pastels with pastels, brights with brights, and you can mix any colours – the wilder the better! Don't forget clashing tights! Or go for a big bold print if you really want to stand out (even better: printed dresses have so much going you don't need to worry so much about adding accessories).

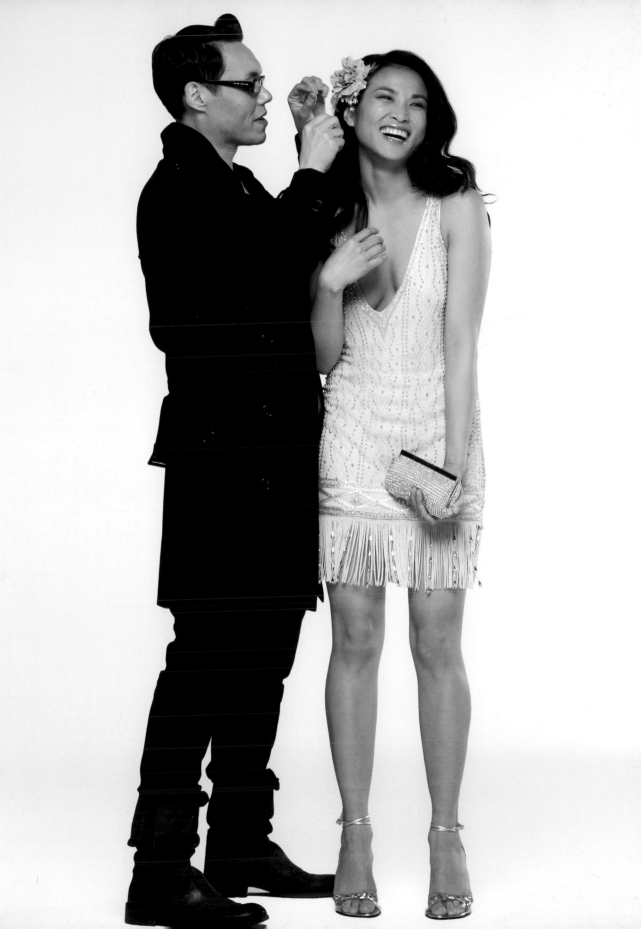

And seeing as first impressions count, how about a dress with a striking silhouette that makes an instant style statement? From a perky prom dress to a loose and cool sack dress, a one-shoulder asymmetric style or a simple A-line shirt dress, a funky cut will cut out having to think too hard about what to wear!

For sexy dates and dinner parties, why not find an outfit with some flirty detailing? Ruffles, tiers, pleats, fringing or ruching all add fun and femininity; the perfect pretty top to wear to dinner, or for cocktails, and you'll love the way they move on the dance floor!

For the office party, the point is to show your co-workers the off-duty you. Adding some fabulous accessories to your outfit will showcase your out-of-work personality. Big bold pieces really make a statement; a corsage, large clutch bag, or a chunky belt will turn heads. And how about a funky trilby to let everyone know you've arrived?

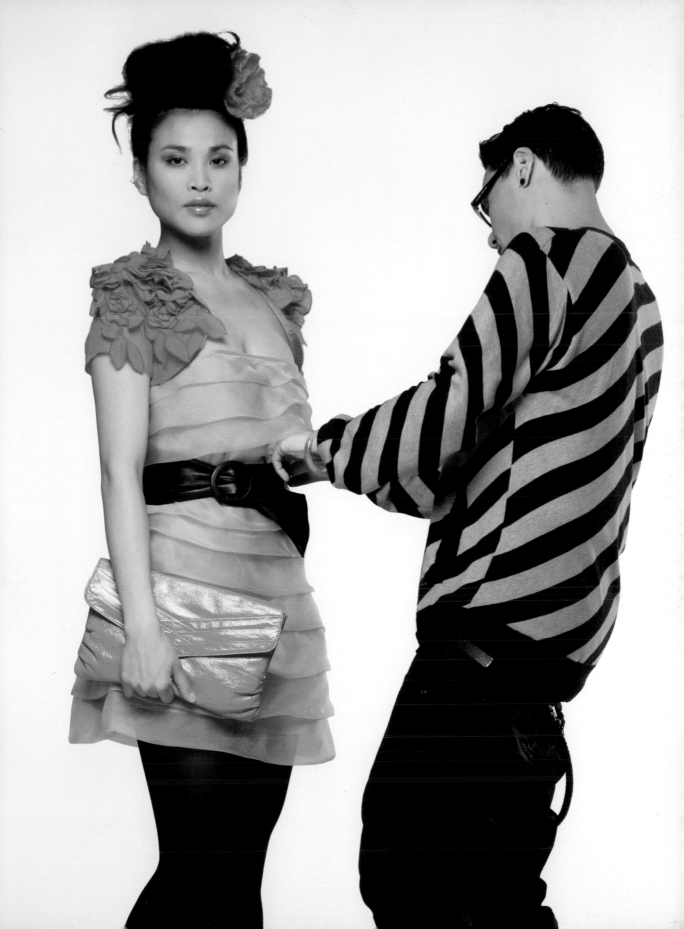

For posher parties, nothing says full-on glamour like a floor-length gown! This is about as formal as it gets fashion-wise. Sometimes the best way to show off your gorgeous body is to cover it all up, head to toe, and making your outstanding outline the focus. And don't think a maxidress has to be demure. Just work a plunging neckline with that plunging hemline; a halter-neck maxi dress is flattering and foxy. And if you love your legs and don't fancy full length, why not go the other way, and flash those pins in a suitably precious-looking embellished dress.

So I'm inviting myself over to yours to create some outfits that celebrate your gorgeousness. And, lady, this invitation is strictly BYOB (Bring Your Outstanding Booty).

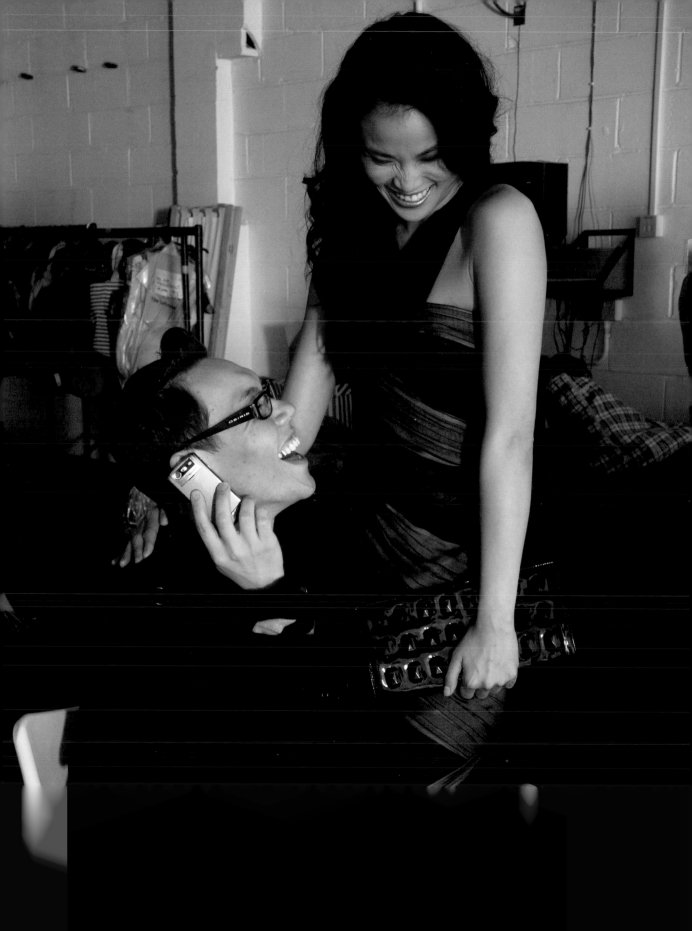

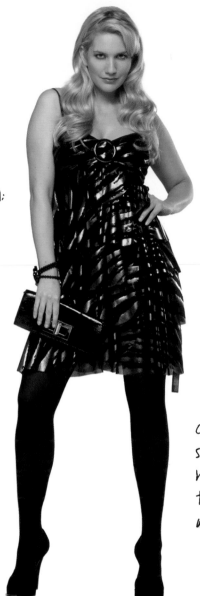

Black doesn't have to be plain; a shiny printed fabric like this is eye-catching and will keep people looking at your fabulous bod!

Opaque tights will stop your shorter hem from feeling too sexy; great for a work do.

THE LBD (little Bold Dress)

The little black dress is a classic: one dress and you've got your whole gorgeous going-out look made! We love that! So it's all about the special-to-your-dress details, like the foxy tiered layers here, which will really add interest and movement to your look (great for shaking your sexy booty on the dance floor).

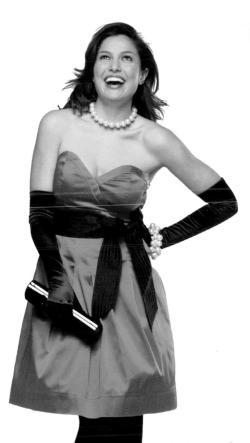

Add a gathered skirt
underneath your dress to
give it extra volume.

Desperate(-ly Sexy) Housewife

This is your Fifties domestic goddess look; very Desperate Housewives. A prom-style dress like this is almost cupcake cute with its sweetheart neckline and bow sash. By mixing tongue-in-cheeky touches like long gloves and pearls with more modern black opaque tights and killer heels, you'll bring this out of the Fifties and bang up to date.

Honey, it's time to leave work at your desk, leave the kids with a babysitter and slip those feet into some dancing shoes!

An evening of laughing constantly with your mates – over food, a film or a bottle or two of something cold – is just the ticket for making the cares of the week fly right out of that window. And no matter what you do, there's nothing like feeling fabulous from the outset to make any night out amazing; you'll always have a good time when you know you're looking good.

So now it's time to assemble a show-stopping going-out number. Dressing for a night out isn't difficult, and by working some bold accessories or a little sparkle into the mix, you can have a going-out outfit in super-quick time.

So let's shop till we drop for a night on the tiles, girlfriend! Let's get this party started!

A night out, my gorgeous, is just what uncle Gok ordered!

HOLIDAYS

Relaxed, sassy and easy-to-pack

- tan leather accessories and wooden jewellery look boho cool
- a strapless top means a strapless tan
- a maxi dress is body flattering and beats the heat

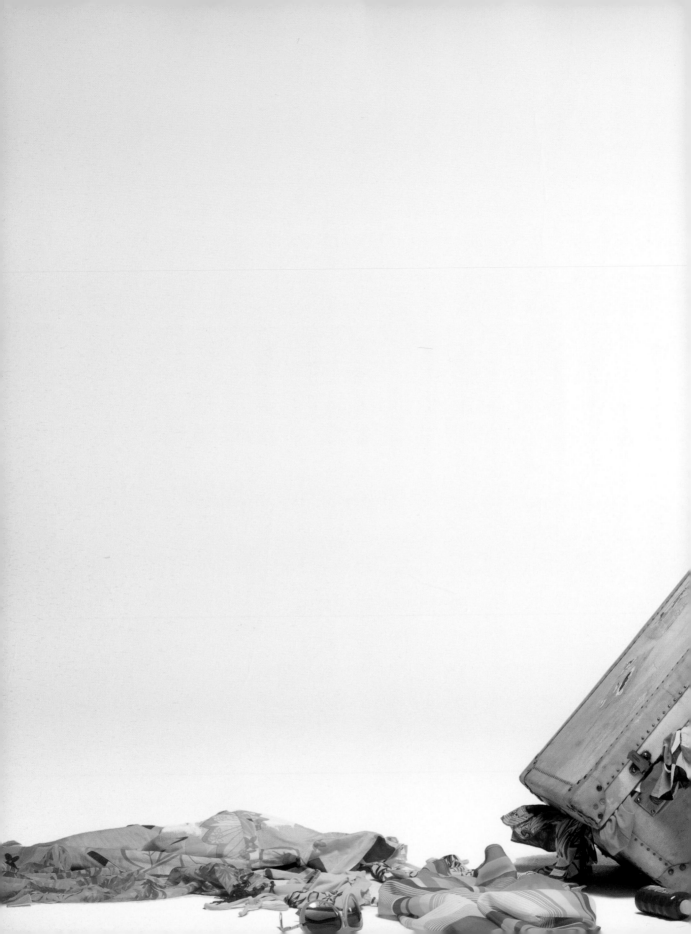

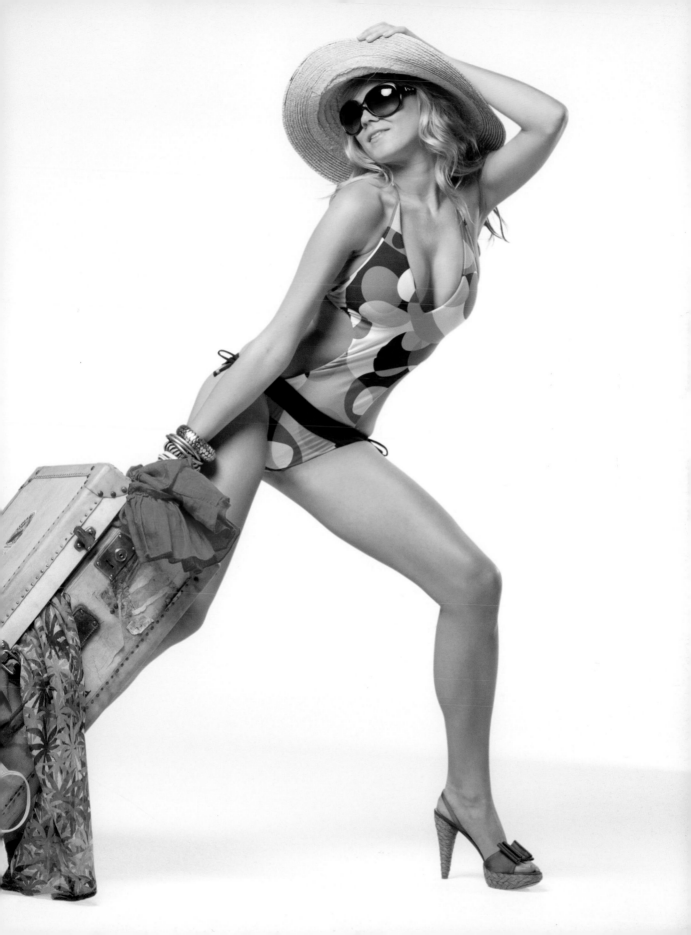

Aaaand … relax. You've earned it. This is your time to get away from it all. To enjoy some sunshine, take in a change of scenery, do whatever you like (or nothing at all), and remember who you really are, gorgeous girl.

PACKING

Don't let those budget airlines' luggage restrictions cramp your style, beach babe! Believe me, it is possible to pack an awesome wardrobe, without being charged for excess baggage.

Your No. 1 top tip to stop you over-packing: trying your outfits on before you pack. Sure, that takes time (but also helps build a nice bit of vacation anticipation!). And it'll save you stuffing your suitcase with things you'll never wear. And think about what you might be doing when you get there – sightseeing? Hiking? Dancing on a yacht?

I like to pack each day's outfit(s) in a separate plastic bag. That way, I don't have to worry when I'm there. Plus, all the layers of plastic cut down on wrinkling.

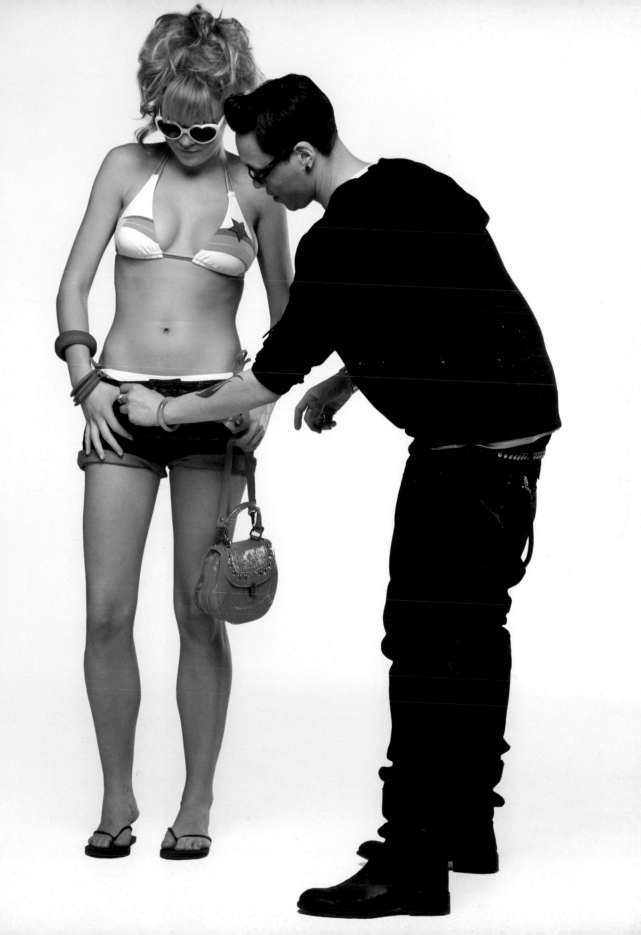

If you plan before you go, when you're on holiday you can forget about your clothes. Which means more time sipping sangria in the sun, and less time working out which shoes go with each outfit. Let the sexy locals think about what you're wearing instead!

ACCESSORIES

Take a maxi bag as your hand luggage. A big beach bag doesn't just store all your stuff, it makes you look smaller in comparison. Then just pack a smaller evening bag, keeping shoes and accessories in the same colour-scheme. Neutrals will work with all your clothes — tan leather accessories and wooden jewellery look boho cool with summer colours, or choose metallics like gold and silver with matching jewellery to up that glamour factor.

Baggage allowance alert: shoes are heavy! For a week's holiday, you probably need one pair you can walk in, like plimsolls or ballet pumps, and some wear-with-anything heels for evening. Then add as many flip-flops and flat sandals as you like — they're much lighter.

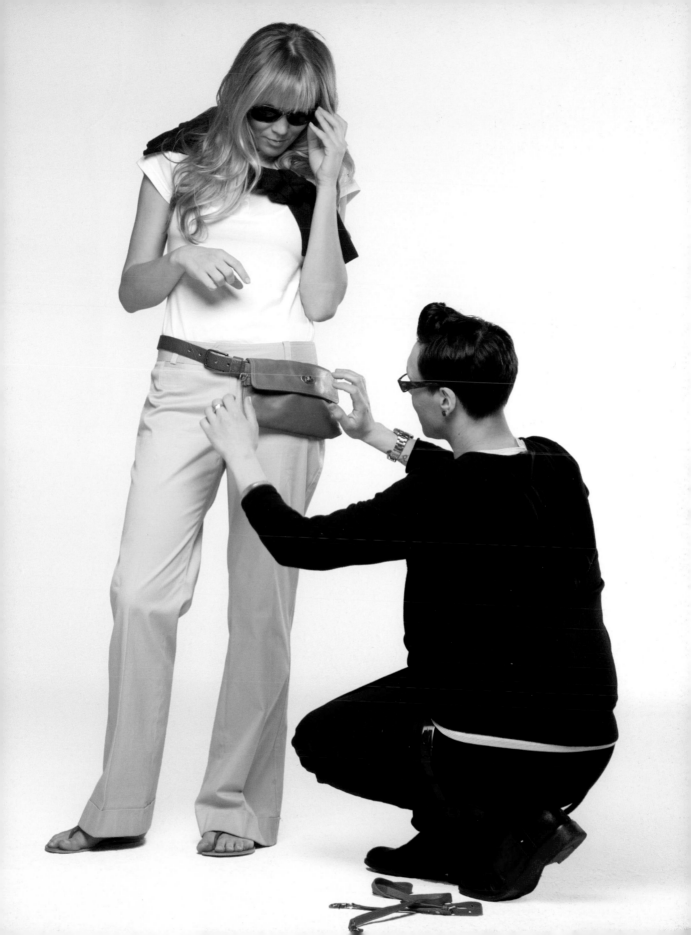

Aside from the poolside waiter in your resort, a scarf will be your best friend on holiday. Shawls, wraps and sarongs take up no space or weight in your case, and are endlessly versatile (see my genius halterneck sarong dress in this chapter!). Tie them around your head, shoulders, hips, chest and neck. In fact, its practically a holiday wardrobe in itself!

HOLIDAY BEAUTY

- Switch to tinted moisturizer – your usual foundation will be too heavy in the heat.

- Start applying that gradual-tan body lotion a week before you go.

- Pack tiny tubes of hot oil treatment; your hair will dry out in the sea and sun.

- Precision-pluck those eyebrows then just wear mascara and tinted lipsalve for the beach.

- Of course you'll be wearing your maximum SPF sun lotion (sunburn wastes tanning time!), but take some fake tan too for those annoying strap marks, and okay, red patches; it's Photoshop in a bottle.

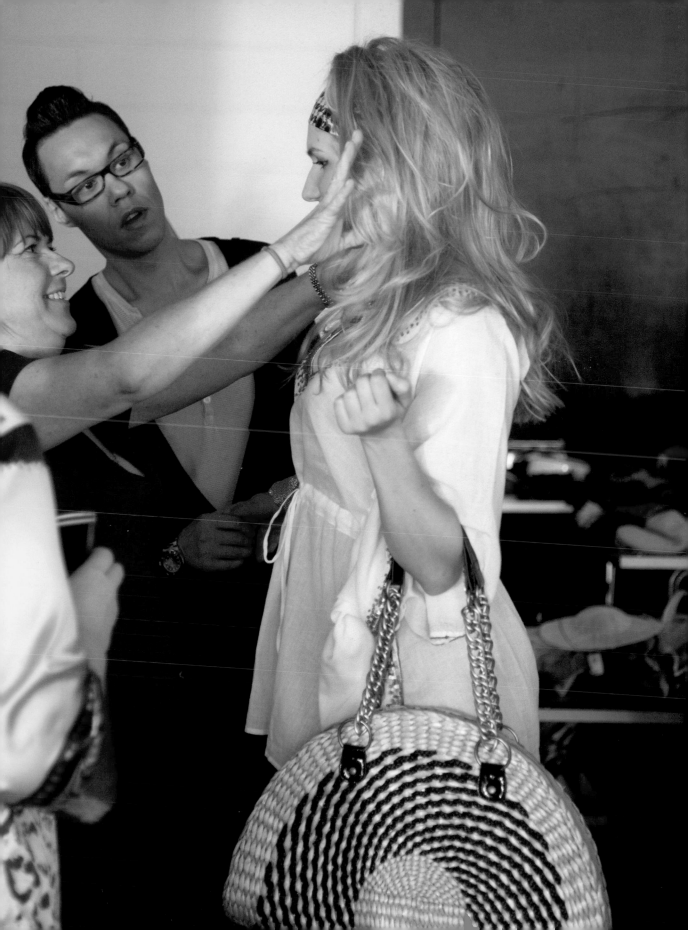

COLOUR

Nothing looks better in sunlight (aside from a margarita) than colour. This is your chance to shine. Nothing will create the illusion of a tan quicker than soft bright colours like turquoises, corals and lilacs. And don't forget, colours that can look harsh at home, like sunshine yellow, will seem softer in the sun. So break out those brights, rainbow babe.

PRINTS

If you don't feel confident putting a colourful outfit together, prints are the answer. Even the simplest patterned dress or bikini can make your outfit look more creative than it is! And nothing, but nothing, screams summer like fresh, flirty florals.

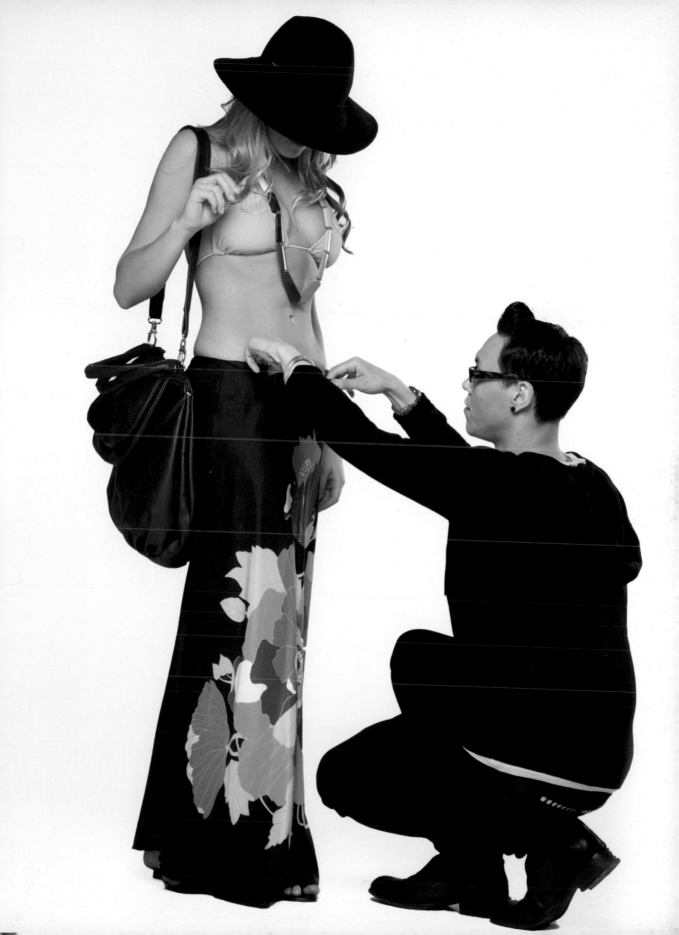

BATHERS

I never understand why curvy girls are beach shy! There is nothing more glamorous than a curvaceous babe in a one-piece. A fitted bather will flatter your foxy figure, and is seriously fashionable right now. Minimizing 'miracle' suits contain micromesh to draw you in in all the right places. Ruching will hide any beach bulges, and for extra inch loss, add a skinny belt to emphasize your tiny waist.

BIKINIS

Your beautiful body is unique. And you're going to need swimwear that does that body justice! Chances are, you're not going to be an off-the-rack size all over (and I love that about you; who wants to be average?), which means choosing a bikini that can be mixed and matched to maximize all of your oh-so-special proportions, with different sized tops and bottoms.

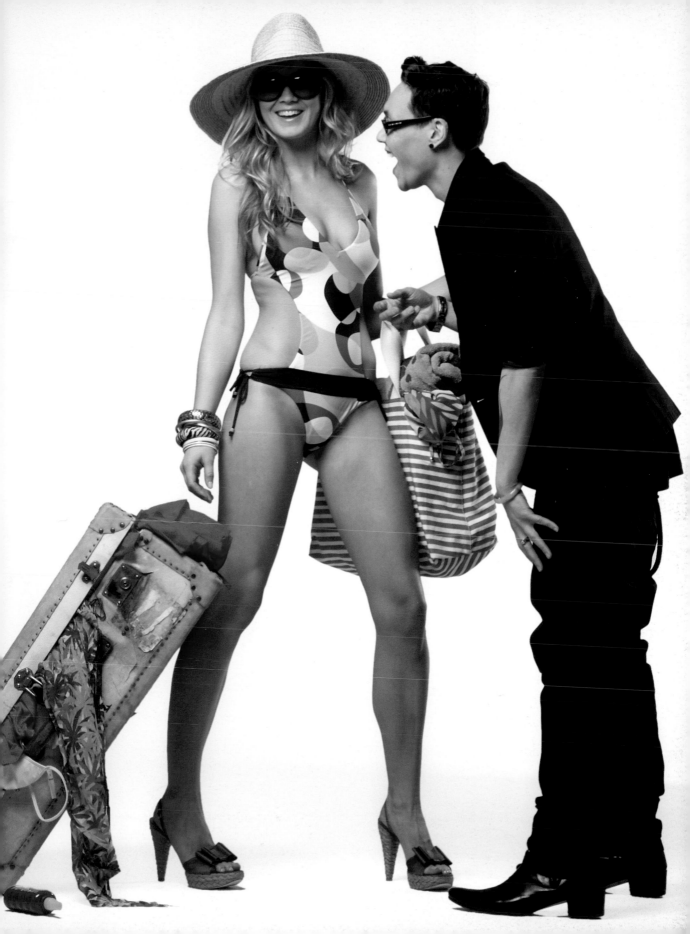

For my ladies with a yummy tummy, don't worry. A bikini doesn't have to be all about your belly, a tankini – with a vest style top – combines body coverage and beach chic; you can still flash some flesh without the muffin tops.

Triangle tops boost those boobs, and tie-sided briefs will add where-did-they-come-from? curves for my skinny minx.

Sexy high-cut briefs will lengthen the pins of even my least leggy ladies. Sex on legs!

Your perfect prints will even out your proportions; for my curvy girl, keep prints big and bold. Adding a darker-coloured print to a plain piece will make the area seem smaller, adding a lighter-coloured print will make the area seem bigger.

Vertical stripes are slimming, the perfect briefs for pears; and horizontal stripes will broaden your curves, giving you an even weenier waist. Wowsers!

But now, it's time to get on the case with what to pack in that case ... read on!

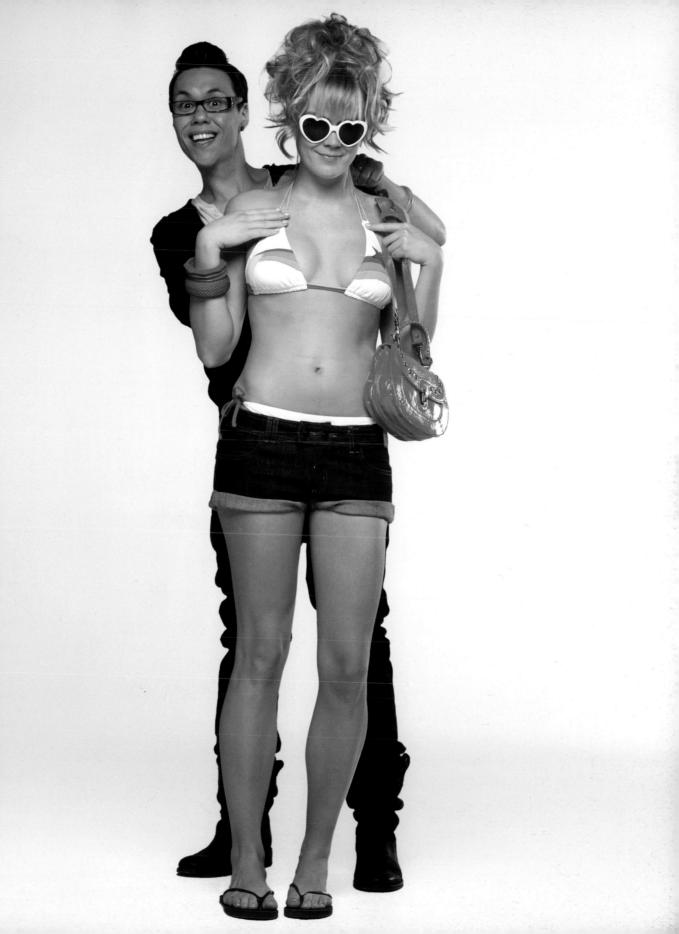

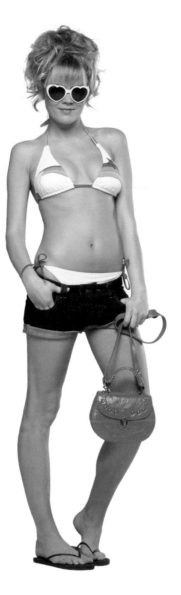

A multicoloured bikini is easy to accessorize, just pick out any of the colours — like this red swing bag.

A large fringey bag carries the western theme through.

California Girl

Who wants to take things seriously on the beach? Now even my English roses can get some Californian cool. A cartoony white bikini, crazy glasses, and denim hotpants all show your young and fun side; I want to come on holiday with you!

Daisy Duke

Yee-ha! Cowgirl is a seriously hot beach look for you, and all you have to do is add a hat! The straw Stetson is your ultimate beach accessory; it's cool and sexy, and offers great sun protection. What's not to like?

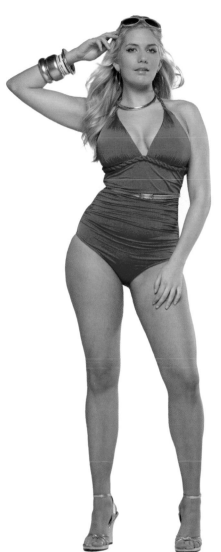

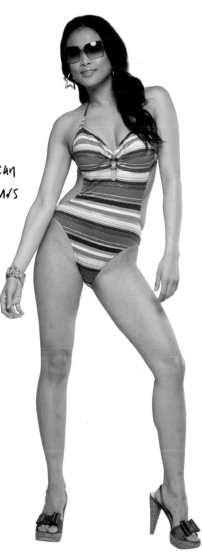

Your sunglasses can highlight colours in your swimsuit; like the gold frames and brown lenses here – slick!

Add glamour with matching gold accessories: big bangles, strappy sandals and a (waist-defining) skinny belt.

Marilyn Monroe

Ready for your close up? Too right! You're going to look like a Fifties movie star in this retro-style bather. Show your super-sophisticated side in a swimsuit dressed up with accessories you usually reserve for evening!

Hip-hop Honey

Guess what? A cut-out swimsuit can be every bit as sexy as a bikini. This is your hip-hop look, honey; just add a 'bling' gold bracelet, sexy heels and a little urban attitude and you'll be the hottest babe on the beach.

loose sleeves will give your outfit a breezy elegance, especially with bangles or a bracelet.

white and gold are easy to match, look great with a tan and add instant glamour to your outfit.

Kaftan Queen

Let's face it, not everyone wants to play beach origami with a sarong! Traditional kaftans like this are cut in a simple square shape, but when you throw it on, it's fabulously drapey, making you look foxy and floaty. A cinched waist and low, open neck will skim your tummy and focus on your sexy curves.

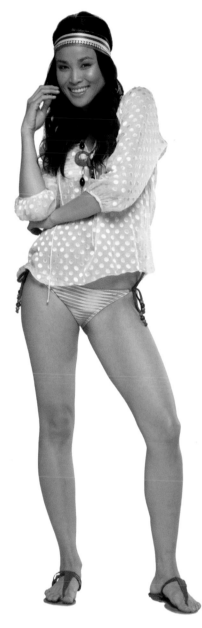

Gok's sneaky style tip
A light-coloured headband adds a touch of summer to dark hair.

Yes, you can mix prints - and it's even easier if one of the colours matches.

Far out and Funky

Lady, let's see those lovely legs! You can use a pretty smock or tunic top from your summer wardrobe on the beach, as a dressier alternative to throwing on a sarong.

Details like a light or sheer fabric and three-quarter sleeves work really well. Who says that covering up on the beach can't be sexy?

wear it another way: You will look
so chic in this skirt for evening
(pack a vest top in that beach
bag). You can even wear it as a
strapless dress!

Hip Hippy

Sarongs will be your best friend on holiday. But as a slinky alternative, a maxi skirt will showcase your sexy midriff and hips. This is your rich hippy look. A wider brim will give your sunhat a bit of Seventies style. The funky lovebeads necklace puts the focus on your gorgeous torso and a maxi bag makes you look even teenier.

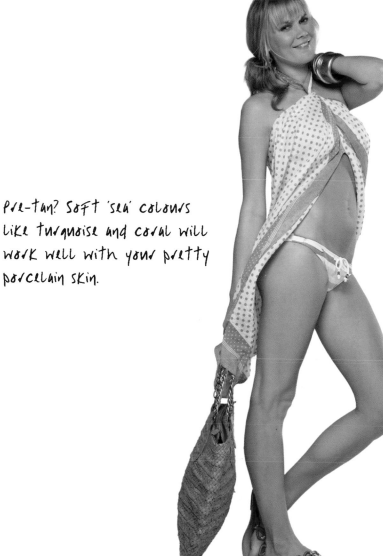

Pre-tan? Soft 'sea' colours like turquoise and coral will work well with your pretty porcelain skin.

Sassy Sarong

Girlfriend, you're now enrolled for Gok's Sarong Masterclass! For this sophisticated halterneck look: hold two corners of the fabric, swapping hands three times to twist, and then tie around the back of your neck. This style will still show off your lovely tanned shoulders (and a cheeky flash of bikini brief).

A large-brimmed sunhat is a movie star classic; it keeps all eyes on you while also keeping you mysteriously out of sight; add large sunglasses for extra movie-star style.

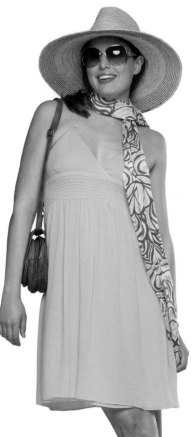

A side-tied, long hanging scarf shaves inches off your hips.

Bags with adjustable straps are endlessly versatile; wear across the body or shorten to wear under the arm.

Sunshine Chic

Nothing says sunshine like a clear bright yellow dress. And yes, you can wear this confident fresh colour, my English rose – if necessary just add a complexion-flattering scarf, with yellow in the pattern, closer to your face.

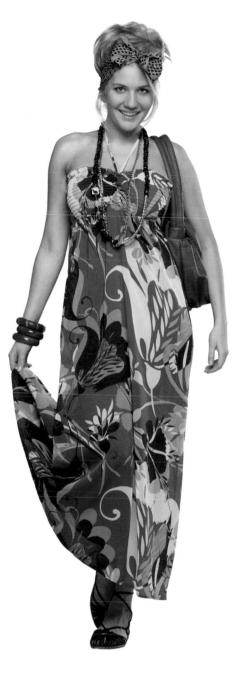

Tan leather accessories and wooden jewellery work well with summer colours and keep all eyes on the dress.

Tropical Beauty

A bold colourful all-over print is a great style statement, and will keep you cool in the summer heat. This is your ultimate head-to-toe outfit-in-one, an ankle length dress is instantly slimming, easy-peasy and glamarama! How much do you love me?

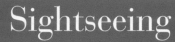

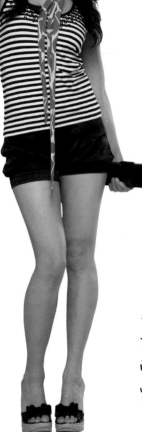

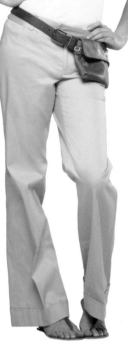

Bangles and a clutch are a great combination for dinner; keeping all your accessories action on the table top.

Flip-Flops flash a bit of flesh, even if it's just below your ankle.

French Beach Chic

Simple basics, like a stripy vest or black shorts, can work for evening spiced up with sexy accessories. You could even pack these in your beach bag and swap flip-flops for heels if you head straight from the beach to the bar!

Euro-preppy

Sometimes the simplest ideas are the best! The preppy look is classic and classy (and not everyone wants to sightsee in hot-pants!) This look suits all body shapes as the polo shirt and chinos come in so many different cuts.

Not all summerwear has to be skintight! Relaxed shorts balance a loose top, but still give you slinky hips.

Flirty Florals

How can your avoid those pesky strap marks? Your solution is simple, my bronzed goddess – strapless styles mean a strapless tan! A loose cotton top like this will keep you cool in the heat (as well as showcasing your saucy shoulders) and make your hips look teeny in contrast (bonus!). And floral prints will keep you looking fresh and pretty.

Tops with a predominantly vertical pattern like this will elongate and slim your body.

This super-ornate bag and necklace mirror each other style-wise.

PUFFBALL BABE

Prom dresses are so versatile, wear them with serious heels and you're black tie formal. With sandals, it's your cute sundress for day, or your foxy cocktail frock for a holiday night out (heels in the heat aren't really an option). A puff ball skirt will instantly give you a weeny-waist.

Simply Slinky

Girlfriend, I know you love your magic underwear, but on a hot night, control spandex is as welcome as a mosquito bite. An empire line top with a loose hem will skim your yummy tummy. And a top with an asymmetric hem will be super-flattering on those gorgeous hips.

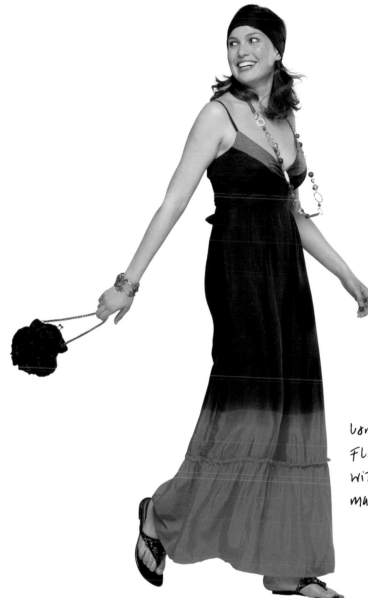

GoK's sneaky style tip
Balance out those
beautiful bangers
with a flounce hem.

Longer necklaces are
flattering and funky
with your foxy
maxi dress.

Sexy Señorita

A ruffly flamenco-style dress is a fabulously romantic holiday look for you. Black is super-slimming and will give your evening outfit a Mediterranean-style sophistication. Maxi dress styles are fitted to the smallest part of your hot bod, then cool and floaty to the floor (nice). Flat embellished evening sandals like these will complete your sexily relaxed look. And you can add a flower for real flamenco style. Olé!

Accessories

Decisions, decisions … It's always a dilemma deciding what to pack and what not to pack, but any of these holiday accessories will be worth the space they take up in your case!

1 A sunhat with a deep crown (like a Stetson) will add instant height to elongate your body.

2 Make your bikini even sexier – just add a long necklace (but beware: metal might burn!).

3 A pretty headscarf will add a flash of summer colour to dark hair.

4 Can't kick your heel habit? Chunkier raffia soles look right for the beach.

5 Nude-coloured flip-flops keep the emphasis on your outfit.

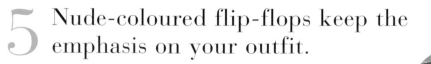

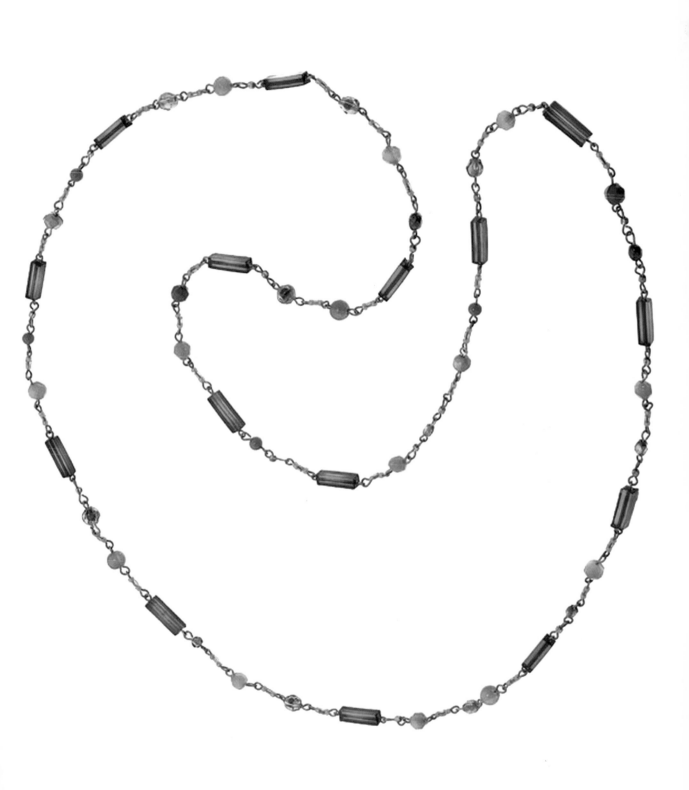

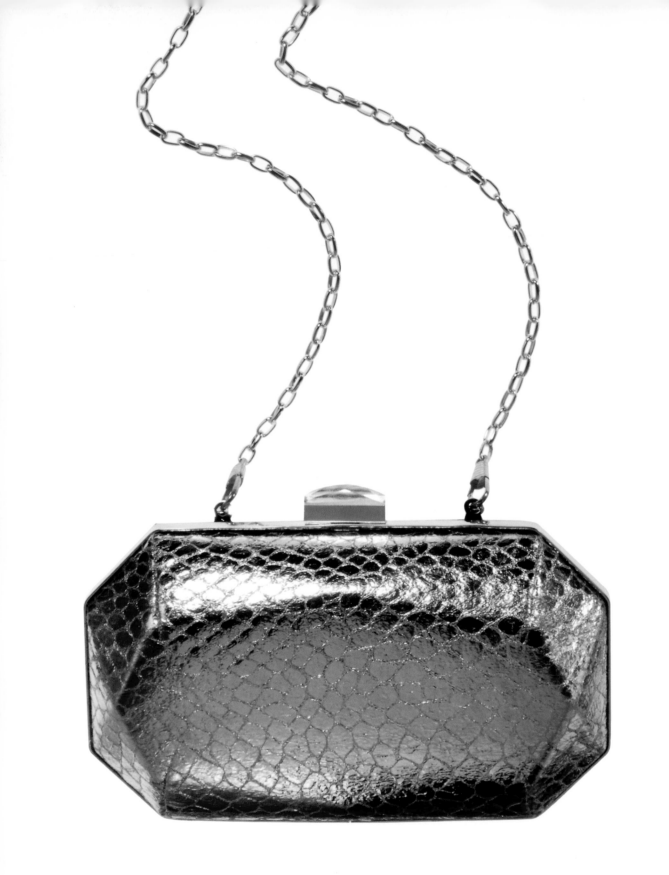

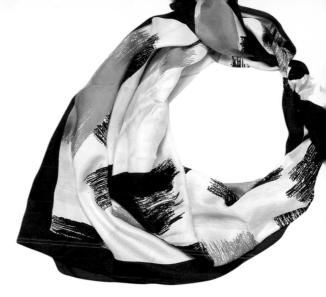

6 Tie a funky headscarf in a bow to restyle your wet-from-the-pool hair in an instant!

7 A belly chain will highlight your sexy waist (muffin tops beware!).

8 A slouchy low-slung maxi bag will give your look a laid-back hippy feel.

9 A hard, structured clutch bag won't get crushed in your suitcase.

10 Ethnic wooden beads will add a bit of boho to your beach outfit.

It won't be long before you're strolling in the sea, lounging on the beach and watching the sun go down with a delicious cocktail in your hand.

Following the style tips in this chapter will be your passport to a no-brainer vacation wardrobe. Because once you've arrived, you won't want to be working hard at looking gorgeous – it just needs to happen! But don't worry, my darling. Whether you're going on a road trip, taking a luxury cruise, or flying on a budget airline, I promise you, your wardrobe is going to be first class!

By clever packing and trying on things before you go, you're going to arrive and find you love everything in your suitcase (now that's what I call a holiday romance!). And let's not forget, the holiday might only last a week or so, but the holiday snaps are going be around for years to come. So remember to pack some SPF (sexy pieces of fashion!)

So now you've just got one stopover en route to that lovely vacation destination – the shops! Let's get out there and buy you some fabulous new holiday-wear to bring out your inner beach babe! Get set to join the jet set!

Girlfriend, I'm so jealous you're going away! Will you pack me in your suitcase?

WEDDINGS

Foxy, formal and photo-fabulous

- a super-chic coat can make a wedding outfit
- experiment with colour for maximum impact
- a wide-brimmed hat adds drama

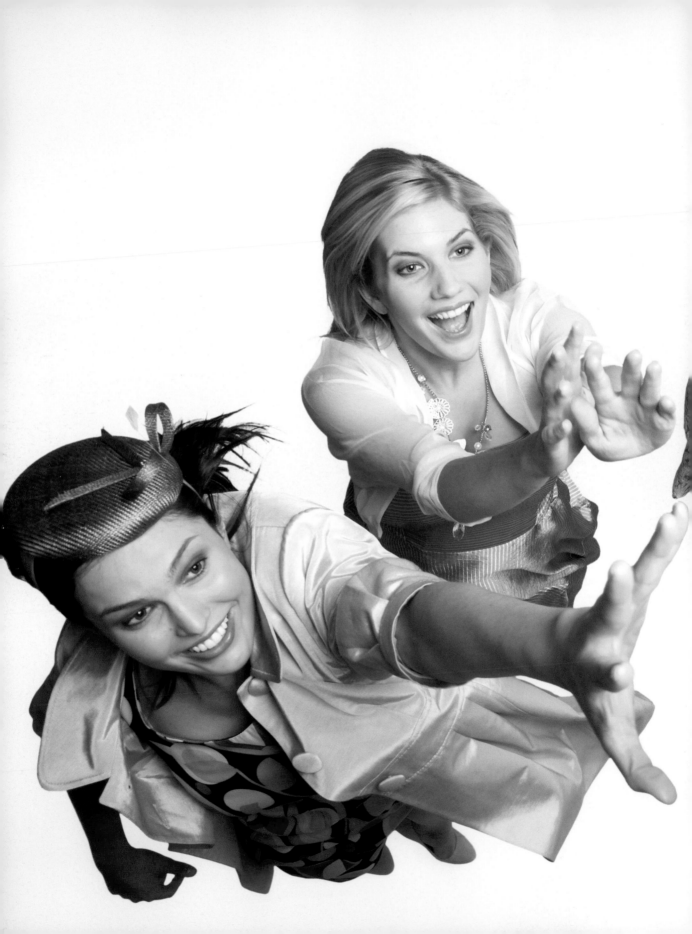

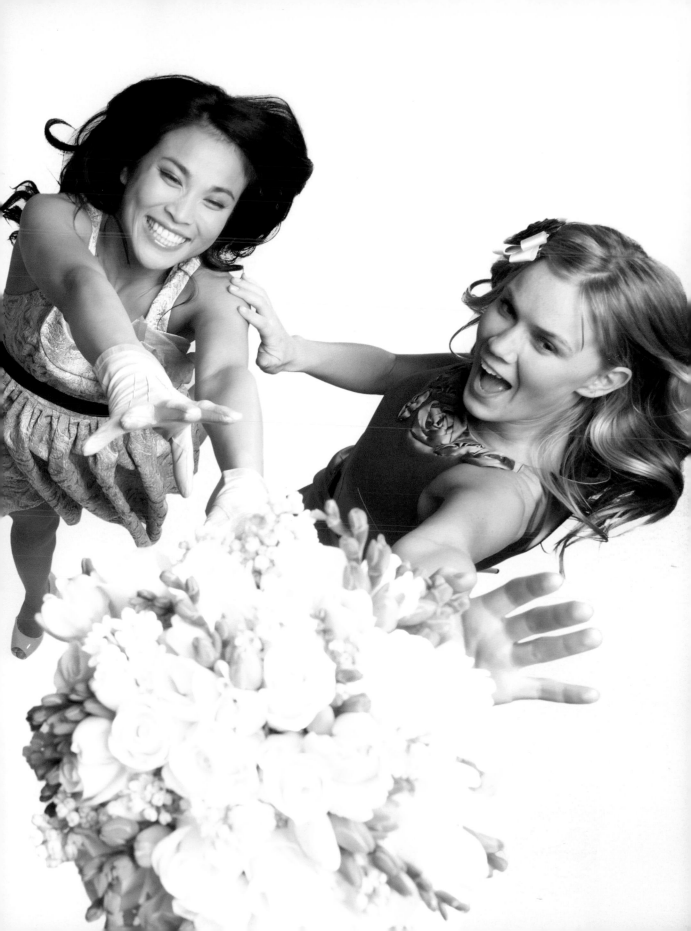

I love weddings! Girlfriend, this is your time to dress to impress. You're not supposed to upstage the bride, but – let's face it – all eyes are going to be on you. Even the groom will be having second thoughts, once he's clocked how we're going to showcase your fabulous outfit. All you have to do is commit to keep Gok's Fashion Vows … For fitter, for foxier, in chicness and in hats …

Wearing colour will draw attention to your beautiful body

Those peach-satin bridesmaids are going to be green with envy. Weddings are the ultimate opportunity to experiment with some complexion-sexy shades. Autumnal berries and purples are easy to mix-and-match in an outfit, and will look sultry on my darker divas, or give fabulous drama to porcelain-pale babes. For sun-kissed skins (and the fake tan-savvy), pale neutral shades also mix well; team with nude shoes and accessories to keep the focus on your fabulous features.

Fashionistas can go for a clash-tastic catwalk look; teaming an above the knee teal dress, with some contrasting claret tights (and matching shoes) will

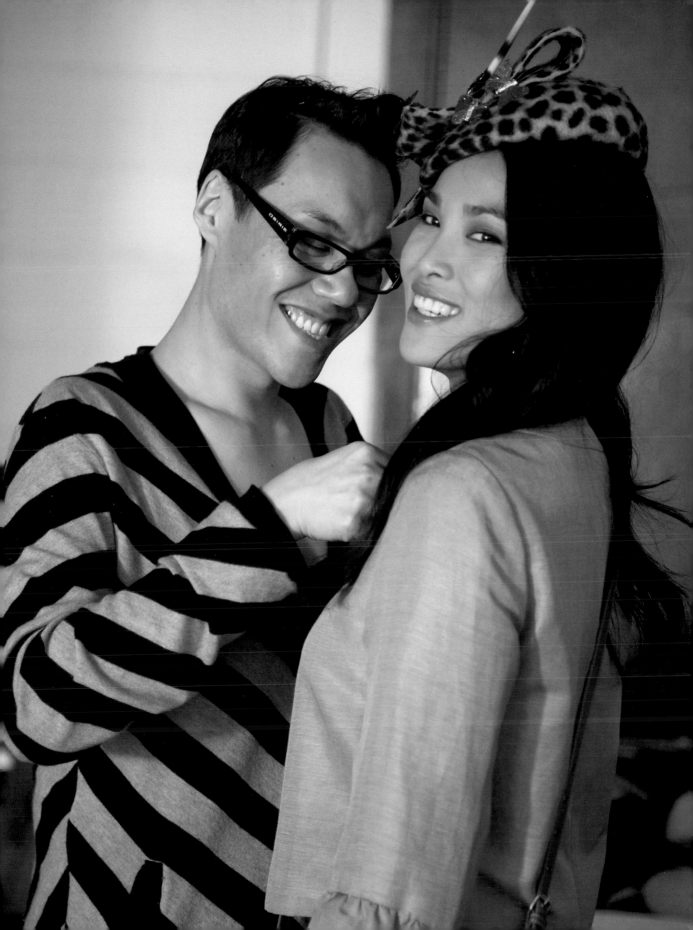

slim the limbs and allow you to strut your sexy stuff. More unusual shades are easy to wear when you choose an entire suit; and carrying the colour through the whole outfit will elongate your beautiful bod – perfect for grabbing the spotlight, and getting you the (male) attention you deserve!

Seriously sexy tailoring will show off your killer curves

Lady, you're going to look amazing in retro suit styles (back in the day, they really knew how to flatter real women's bodies!) A pencil skirt will look sleek but totally smokin' (especially if the hem kicks out to add even more traffic-stopping curves!). Team with the classic, chic-belted, open-neck jacket for your Marilyn Monroe moment (boo boo be doo). Or maybe you're more of a sweet Sixties type; a chic-patterned swing-style jacket with three-quarter sleeves will make you look like a Hitchcock-heroine ice maiden, and a slim, below-the-knee-length skirt will lengthen those luscious legs. Or go Sexy Seventies in a sophisticated trouser suit with a fitted jacket and fabulous flared trousers.

You're going to look HOT when the temperature rises.

Summer weddings are your opportunity to shine. Just follow Gok's style slogan K.I.S.S. (keep it simple, sexy). I don't want you to have to think about anything except topping up your fake tan, so I'm going to find you the perfect dress that's going to do everything for you; an outfit-in-one!

With dresses, it's all in the detailing, so listen up:

- Go for big bold prints to give you instant glamour.

- Slink your bod into an empire line maxi dress for a breezy boho moment (perfect in the heat).

- Throw on a foxy cocktail dress to keep you looking confidently chic; a wide prom skirt will showcase your sexy legs, and a halterneck gives a glimpse of your gorgeous bare back and shoulders.

- A bow detail below the bust adds a cute retro touch (as well as keeping attention on your beautiful bangers – quite right too!).

- Tiers, ruffles or flounces will give you a flirty femininity and will move like a dream on that dance-floor.

A super-chic coat can make a wedding outfit. And it's the first thing anyone sees when you make your entrance, during the service, and, of course, in all those wedding photos. And no one needs to know that you're hiding a va-va-voom outfit for hitting the dance-floor later (you don't want to distract the vicar during the vows).

And just as important, jumping into one piece will get you to the church on time – brilliant! Your entrance-making outerwear will be turning heads.

Something old

The classic three-quarter-length single-breasted A-line coat, with an open neckline and a waistband that hugs and highlights that tiny waist will have you hearing wolf-whistles. Or choose a neat, foxily-fitted shape that finishes above the knee.

Something neu(tral)

A cream or very pale coat will work wonders with any wedding outfit, and will still look fabulous year after year.

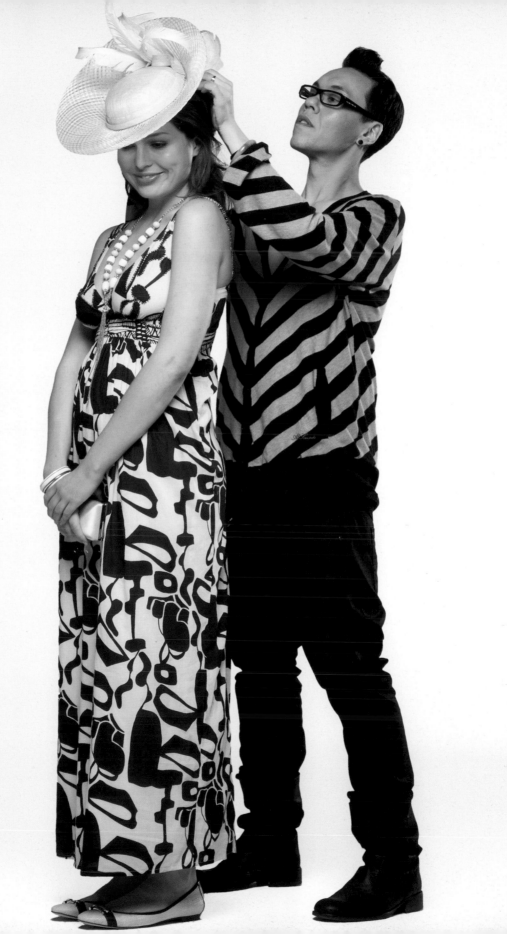

Something bolero

You don't have to cover up in a full-length coat! Keep it all about your dress in a cropped bolero, shoulder shrug, or even a little knitted jacket.

Something blue

Choose a coat in an attention-seeking shade so everyone notices you arriving in style.

And finally ...

If you hate hats, hold your (bare) head high; chic hair is always a great look.

Trust me, trousers are allowed; a dressy trouser suit looks seriously sophisticated (especially on a luscious English pear).

Black is fabulous, not a faux pas (just don't wear it head-to-toe).

So forget etiquette, and wear whatever makes you feel gorgeous - it's your special day too!

Turn the page for some more of my super-stylish suggestions ...

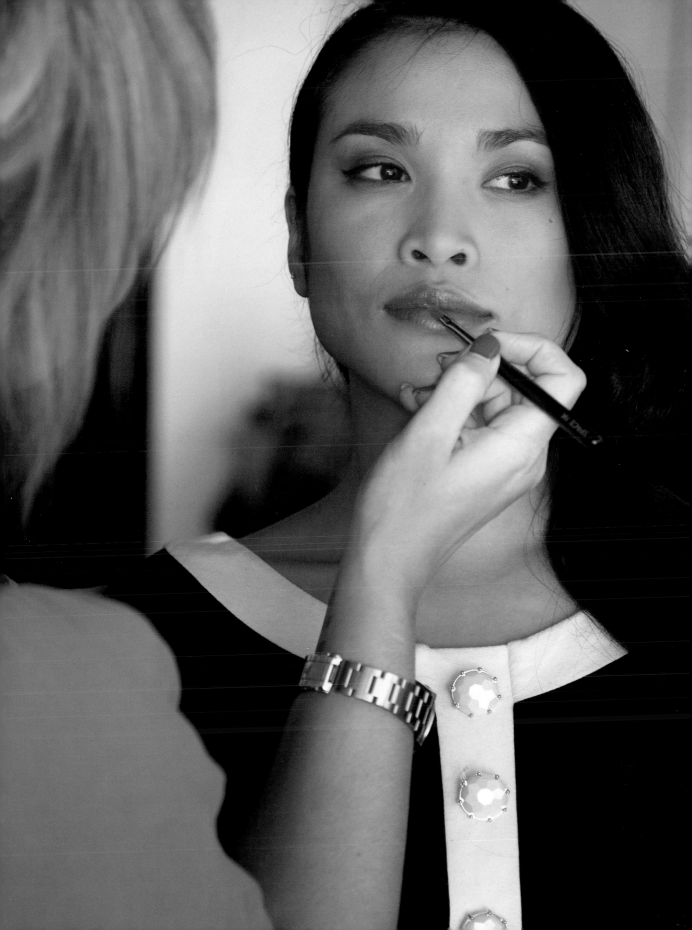

An animal print hat will add even more grrr to your super-sexy ensemble.

Neutral accessories keep the focus on that attention-grabbing suit.

Technicolour Glamour

Weddings are great occasions for you to experiment with colour. Finding a shade that only you can pull off is really going to make you stand out from the crowd.

A mid-length skirt like this might seem difficult to wear, but carrying the colour through with a matching jacket really elongates your beautiful bod!

Show off your elegant arms with some elbow length gloves and three-quarter-length sleeves.

Hitchcock Heroine

Want to be the show-stopping guest at the wedding? Think: Hitchcock heroine; prim but sexy (appropriate for a wedding but will also get you some action). Channel your inner-diva with details like a dramatic wide-brimmed hat or elbow-length gloves. Ladylike accessories like stilettos or a clutch bag will bring out your femme fatale.

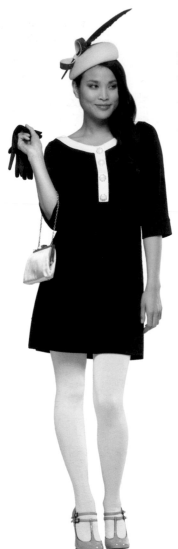

Sweeping your hair to one side is a great way to balance an asymmetrical hat.

Wearing a jacket open to reveal just a narrow column of dress elongates your sexy silhouette.

Parisian Chic

This, my lovely, is your tribute to Coco Chanel! Black and white will give you a little Parisian chic for any event. A simple black dress will always make you look effortlessly stylish (and slim!). Soft-coloured accessories like these add a sophisticated twist.

Foxy Vixen

When you know you look gorgeous in your favourite little black dress, you need to use every opportunity to strut your sexy stuff! Black looks wonderful for weddings, combined with another colour. Add a structured jacket and a matching flirty hat, and you'll be smouldering!

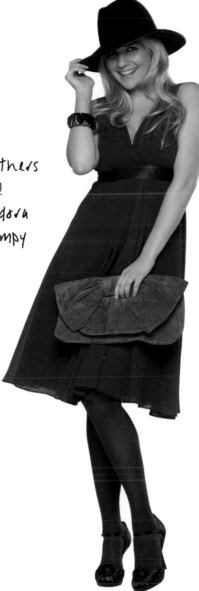

Don't just think feathers for wedding headgear! A felt hat like a fedora could make a very vampy alternative.

Purple Vamp

Guess what, you can still look like a total vamp for those wedding days when the weather can't make up its mind (ah, don't you just love Britain?). Strong, bright colours like purple, red or bright blue will keep you looking confident and stylish come rain or shine (or y'know, both). Your secret weapon: tights! Whip them on or off as the weather dictates ... or when you hit the dance floor!

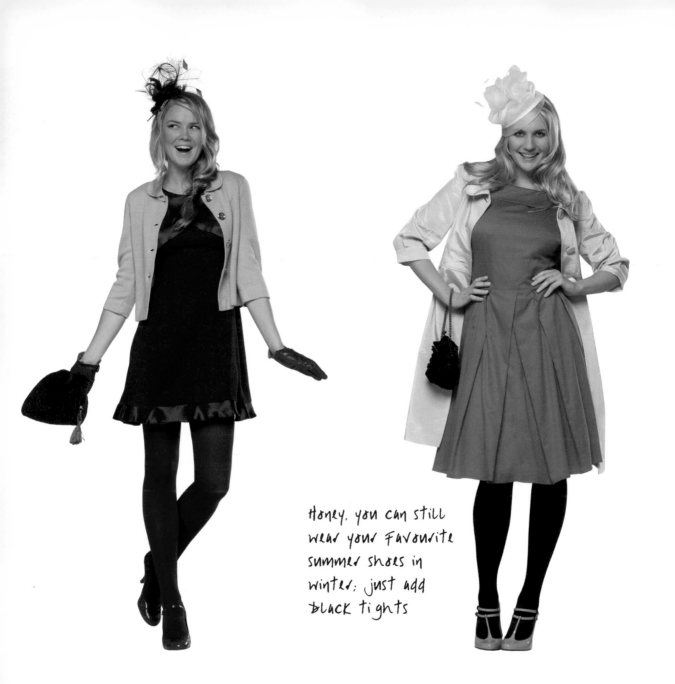

Honey, you can still wear your favourite summer shoes in winter; just add black tights

Flirty Forties

How cute are you? Vintage style dresses like this Forties frock will make you look sweet and flirty. Ditch the tailoring, a little cardigan will give your dress a touch of retro romance.

Ruby Babe

Gorgeous girl, this is your one-stop wedding outfit which has it all going on! Perfect for all my lovely ladies, a knee-length cocktail dress like this sexy scarlet number will never go out of style.

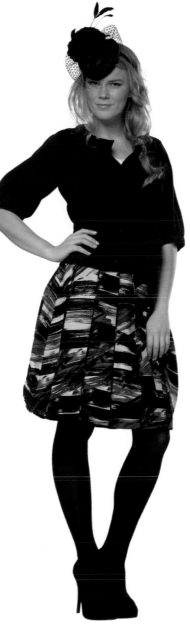

Gok's sneaky style tip
Wider skirts will make your legs look super-skinny (love that!).

With a fabulous full skirt like this, keep the rest of your outfit hugging your foxy figure!

Catwalk Queen

This, my trendy lady, is one look that you can take straight off the catwalk and right down the aisle. An unusual skirt like this patterned bell one will show everyone how fashion forward you are. Which of course you are! Matching it with black will keep your look demure enough for a wedding (and also makes wearing this show-stopping piece oh-so-simple for you!). Gorgeous!

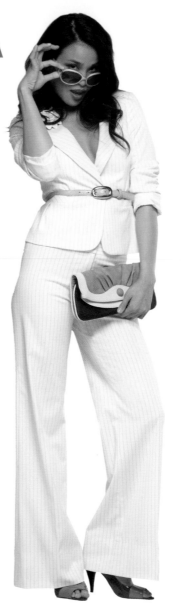

Bold lipstick keeps your face the focus in a white suit.

Yes, you can wear white as a wedding guest (as long as its not a Vera Wang meringue, you little minx).

St Tropez Babe

Sexy lady! The impossibly sleek Bianca Jagger married Mick in a white trouser suit in the Seventies, and now you can try this breezy and glamorous look too. A dressy trouser suit will make you look formal for the church and foxy on the dance-floor. Loose sexy hair will help you exude femininity. Vive la différence!

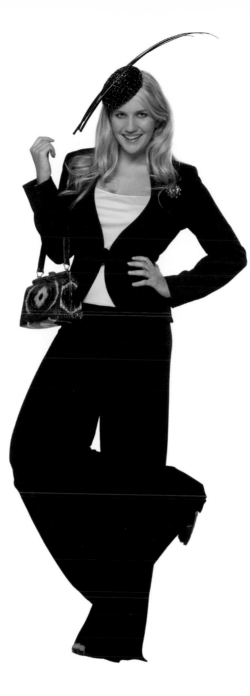

Gok's sneaky style tip
A belted jacket like this will emphasize your fabulous waist.

Black Beauty

Honey, whoever said you can't wear black to a wedding was probably trying to stop turning up looking THIS hot. A black outfit will look fabulously classy on you. A dressier cut, like these wide-legged trousers will give your suit added sophistication. And you can slip a sexy camisole style top underneath the jacket. Wowsers!

Adding one brightly coloured accessory like these fabulous fuschia gloves can give your monochrome look a seriously sassy twist.

Peep-toe detailing can stop black shoes looking too heavy for your light coloured dress!

Prom Princess

A simple prom dress is such a polished look that people will assume you're part of the wedding party! Sticking to one colour for all your accessories is easy on your stress levels and easy on the eye! You'll be stealing the limelight, my princess!

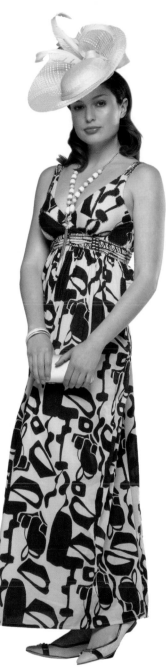

it's easy to accessorize bold prints if you stick to one of the colours.

Floor Length and Foxy

Believe me, girlfriend, you can still stay cool at a tropically hot wedding. Your favourite summer maxi dress will feel breezy and glamorous, simply ditch the flip-flops for more formal accessories like a fabulous hat and an elegant bag.

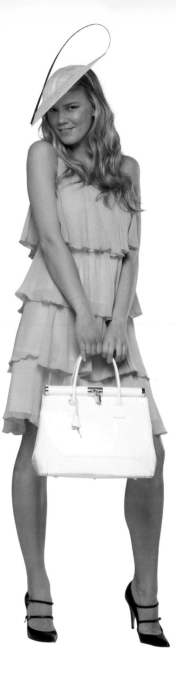

A simple bag and hat help you balance fabulously fussy ruffles.

mint hot chick

A feminine tiered dress like this will keep you looking fresh and pretty at a summer wedding. Light chiffony fabrics work well with girly detailing like ruffles, and after dark, those flouncy layers will come alive on the dance-floor at the reception. You go, girl! Don't feel you have to match ice cream colours head to toe; black and white will give a slick finish to your look.

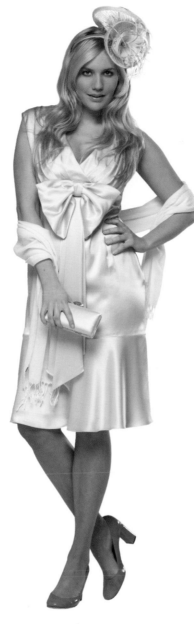

Hat shy? muted tones can stop your head gear looking too wacky.

Gok's sneaky style tip
Neutral shoes lengthen those legs and keep all eyes on your dress

The Glamour Wag

This, my darling, is your all-out WAG-chic look! Forget fashion, this is all about you, and your high voltage gorgeousness. A dress with sexy detailing like this boob boosting bow and figure hugging silhouette will do all the talking for you, and trust me – it's saying all the right things. If you're a single babe, then forget catching the bouquet; in a sassy dress like this you'll be bagging the best man!

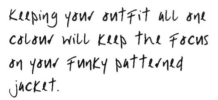

Gok's sneaky style tip
matching trousers and
high heels make your
gorgeous pins go on
forever.

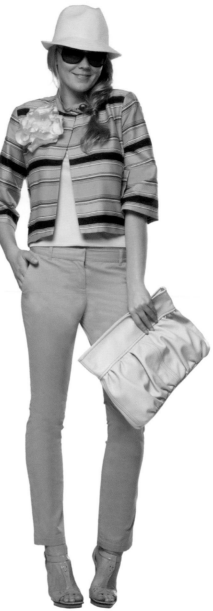

Keeping your outfit all one
colour will keep the focus
on your funky patterned
jacket.

Sassy stripes

Work that look, lady! This funky outfit is perfect for my confident fashionista! You'll look ultra sassy in bold prints like this stripy jacket, and why not top it all off with an extrovert hat like a trilby, while you're at it? On-trend details like the slim cigarette pants, sexy heels, big sunglasses, silk flower and giant clutch bag will give you an edgy but elegant look. You're my style icon!

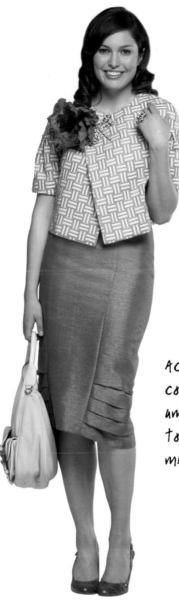

GOK'S
short
help p...
crazily ...
jacket.

Accessories in any
colour will look
amazing with neutral
tones like these
metallics. Easy!

Retro Sexy

Well, ding dong, you Sixties sex kitten! A structured wedding number like this metallic ensemble looks timeless and elegant, while the patterned jacket draws attention up towards your fabulous face and shining hair. All eyes will be on you! By throwing in some ruby red accessories like these shoes and corsage, you'll make this outfit extra special and add some drama to those metallic hues.

Accessories

Weddings are the one place it's acceptable to wear a hat, so go for it, girl! Just choose the hat that will be most flattering to your foxy outfit. And why not say 'I do' to these delectable accessories?

Hats

1 Dark, wide brims create a fabulous sense of drama (oooh, get you); wear with moody hues.

2 Pale, wide brims add sophisticated formality to even your most laid-back summer dress.

3 Neat pill-box hats are a chic option for teaming with retro-sexy suits.

4 Show everyone your cheeky and flirtatious side with a fun feathery fascinator.

5 An angled trilby is funky, but still looks suitably formal for a wedding.

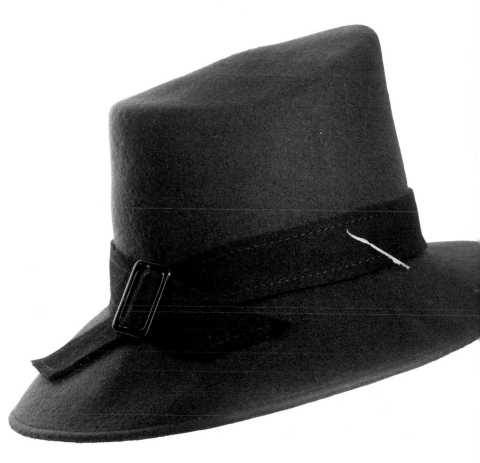

Gloves, bags, jewellery etc.

1 Ornate, vintage-style embellished accessories add something special to a minimalist suit.

2 Nude or metallic accessories will let your dress (and you) shine.

3 A T-bar shoe is very vintage, very sweet (and very cool right now).

4 Ballet pumps can be your chic, dance-till-3am alternative to heels for a wedding.

Fancy looking fashion-savvy? Try some driving gloves to give your outfit an edge.

There's nothing like a wedding to make you feel all warm and glowing inside. After all, where else do we all get together to celebrate something so happy? You're dressed up to the nines and feeling fabulous, you get to see those old friends you haven't seen for years and best of all you can have a good old dance with your mates.

Spending some time on yourself so that you feel 100% gorgeous is the best way to guarantee you'll have a fantastic day to remember. There's no need to worry about who's going to be there when you're looking like a Goddess – all you need to do is sit back and watch as that ex's jaw hits the floor!

There are all too few excuses for you to dress up and show the world your most glamorous, gorgeous self. Whether you're part of the bridal party or not, a wedding is your opportunity to make your star burn brightly. This is your moment in the spotlight and, my luscious lady, I want to see you shine.

It might not be your wedding day, but listen to your Fairy Gokmother and go out and Find the dress of your dreams.

MUMS

On-trend, oh-so you and out-the-door
in ten minutes.

- Boost your body confidence with a bright beautiful print!
- Colourful tights add an easy fashion kick
- You can still wear your favourite biker jacket (even if you can't do it up!)

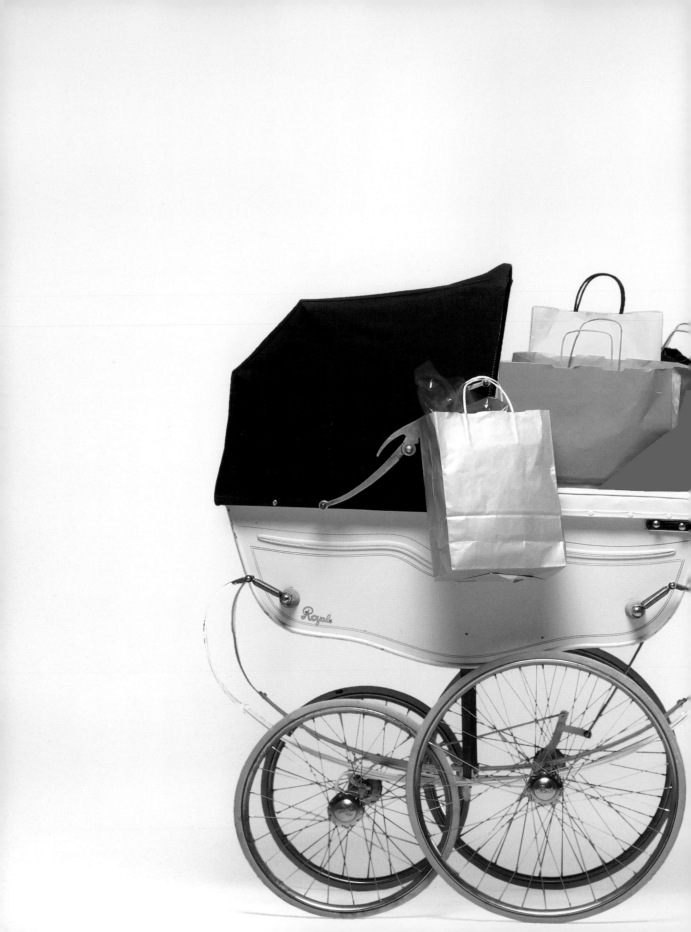

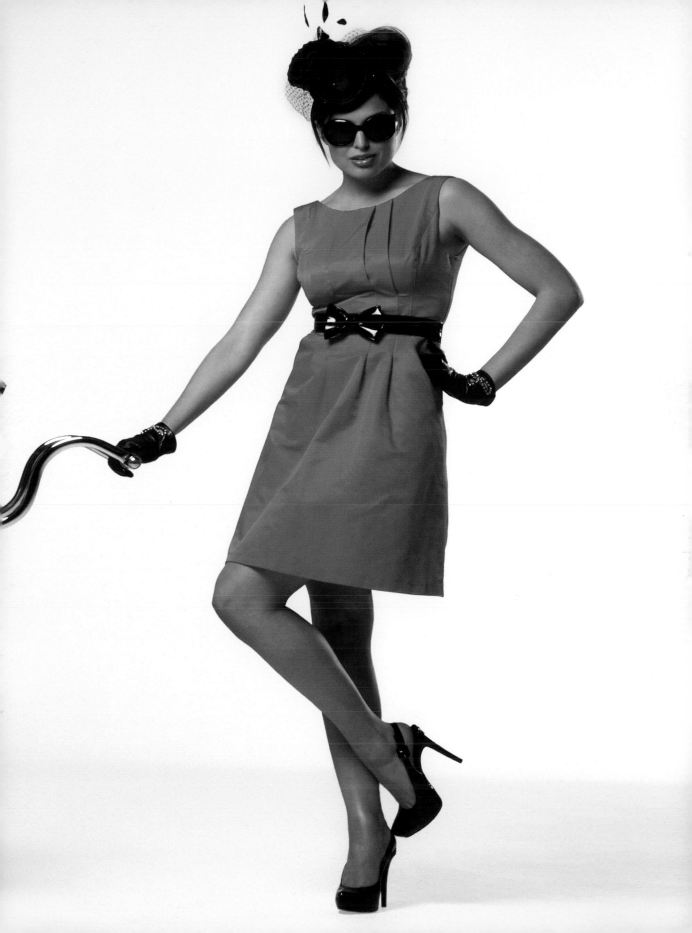

You sexy mother! Okay, I know you sometimes don't feel like that. You probably don't have a lot of Youtime these days, because being a mother is all about being there for everyone else (which really makes you a beautiful woman!).

But I'm now appointing myself your Fairy Gokmother. I'm going to show you some outfits that are so easy to put together that they won't require Youtime or any other time for that matter!

MUMS-TO-BE

You can still be a babe with a baby on board. Maternity might sometimes feel like an alien body invasion, but I can guarantee that everyone else is thinking you've never looked more gorgeous. Of course, you know it's my personal crusade to get women to celebrate their curves; and that includes your luscious baby bump!

Let me introduce you to your two new best friends (no, not the bangers), I'm talking about Mr Elasticated Waist and Mrs Empire Line, you're going to get to know each other very well!

The elasticated waist is all about comfort. You might never have prioritized comfort in your wardrobe before (I love you!) but comfort and support are going to be essential for your growing belly. The empire line is a style that is tightest under your boobs, then drapes over your stomach. It's fabulously stylish and seriously flattering for the bigger belly. And for showcasing those new voluptuous bangers, watch out for v-necks.

It's a brilliant idea to buy some belly-friendly basics; a good pair of jeans with an elasticated waist, some smart trousers, a stretchy pencil skirt, and lots of empire line tunic tops and dresses. Don't make the mistake of thinking 'it's only for a couple of months'. Oh, honey, you wish! My Gokmotherly advice: invest now, so that your capsule wardrobe of brilliant baby-friendly basics can see you through from baby bump to post-baby bulge in style.

Shapes that look great with your new shape

Take it from Gok: cropped skinny jackets that sit on top of your bump totally rock! Women sometimes say 'I won't wear it if it doesn't do up!' but wearing a jacket open to reveal just a narrow column of your dress beneath is a great way to slim your silhouette. Long stretchy skirts can also look amazing, and add a bit of length when you're feeling aaalll about your width!

Is there anything the wrap dress doesn't do? It's still a godsend when you're pregnant. Sleek and superchic, it will work for any occasion, and the sleeveless versions are a great option for summer (remember your arms are going to look super-slim now that you've got bigger curves elsewhere!), and for winter, why not add a luxurious fake fur stole?

And remember, you can still shop on the high street. Many of the outfits in this chapter were bought from 'normal' stores, just a couple of sizes bigger. So don't stop going to your favourite stores.

Post-baby Mum

Maybe you're one of those miracle ladies who fitted right back into their jeans twenty seconds after having a baby. But if you're the other 99.99% of the population, then don't worry!

The loose smock-style top is still huge on the high street, and is super-flattering for bigger tums. Other cuts you can look wonderful wearing include dresses, tunics, empire line, anything maxi, just so long as they skim over your delicious belly.

While darker colours can be slimming, sometimes patterns, graphics and prints are a better option for creating a diversion. And you'll look chic, without looking stuffy.

But forget that belly curve; let's not waste that waist! A smart tailored jacket, with a contrasting belt will focus all attention on your cinched in midsection. And it will look professional and pulled together when you make it back to the office.

On the run Mum

Just because you're a Mum, doesn't mean you can't rock. If you don't usually wear floaty floral frocks or dungarees, why start now? One of my favourite looks in this chapter is Rock-Chick Mum; an edgy, mid-length black jersey pencil skirt, with black ankle boots, a trilby, a cowl neck top, oh, and a leather biker jacket. She looks HOT. And there ain't nothing wrong with that! The point is: don't lose your style.

Here's my top suggestion: if you invest in one piece to sort out your Mum-on-the-school run wardrobe, then get a knock out jacket. You know why? Well, as you may have noticed, your entire life is being lived outdoors; at the school gates, at the playground, in the park, walking home ... A distinctive, colourful coat or indestructible leather jacket will mean you always arrive looking pulled together, even for the dreaded school play. And if you're a car pool Queen go for a shorter three-quarter length jacket, for jumping in and out of that Mum-cab!

Your other essential item, a maxi bag, is bang on trend, and you can also pop in all those assorted Mum essentials.

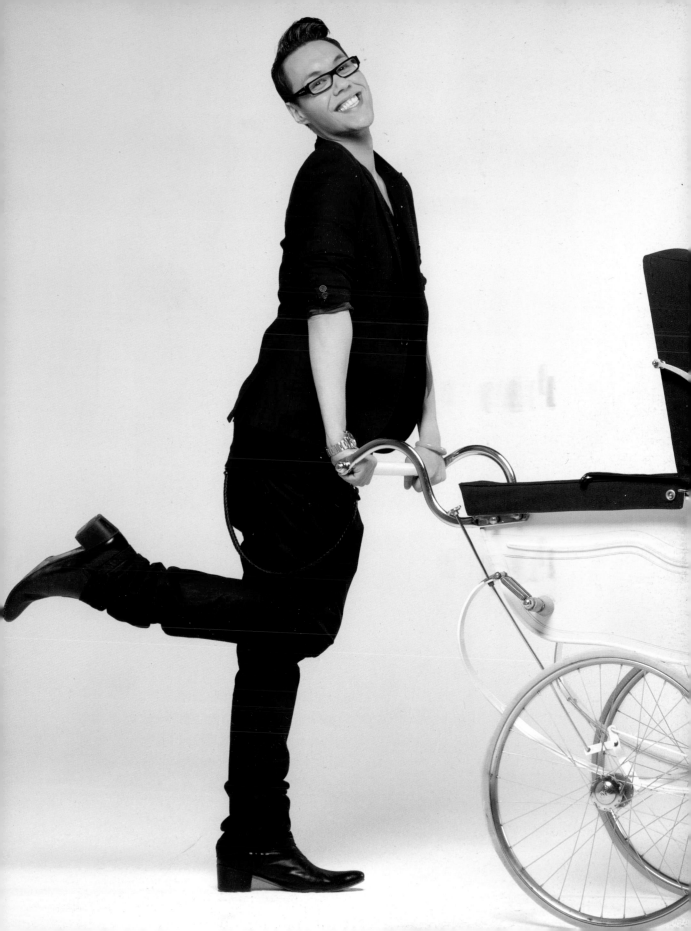

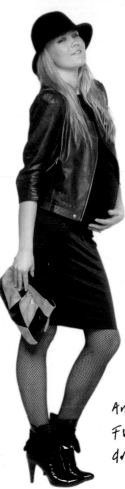

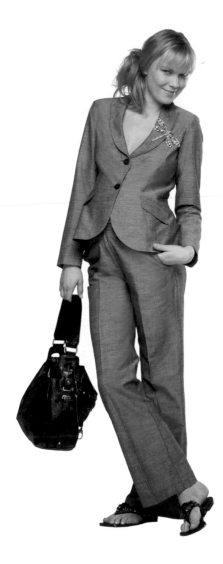

Ankle boots add a funky edge to dresses and skirts.

Rock-Chick Mum

If you've always been a cool rock-chick, you still can be a cool rock-chick when you're a Mum-to-be! So let's have a bit of black lycra; it will streamline your body and showcase your cute little bottom as well as your cute big bump! And you can still wear your favourite leather jacket.

Expecting Exec

If you're used to looking like a slick professional player at work, you don't have to start wearing a formal frock as soon as you're expecting. A longer length suit jacket will accommodate that bump. Buy a jacket with a low cut neckline to elongate the upper body.

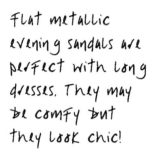

Gok's sneaky style tip
Don't shy away from bold colours when you're pregnant!

Flat metallic evening sandals are perfect with long dresses. They may be comfy but they look chic!

Floor length red dress

How gorgeously glamorous will you be in a floor length dress like this? Maxi dresses are a fabulous option for Mums-to-be! All those pleats can easily accommodate your bump, and best of all, this would be a great piece to invest in that will take you all the way through your pregnancy — and beyond!

A big busy print will also deemphasize your curves, and keeps you in proportion

Your legs will look slimmer than ever in pregnancy; so work those slim jeans!

Sunny Girl

Honey, I'm going to dispel a fashion myth: there's no reason why you can only wear maternity clothes when you're expecting. There are loads of empire line and smock style dresses and tops in the shops, like this funky printed top.

Printy pregnancy

A funky colourful dress like this is endlessly versatile; you can wear it with ballet pumps for day, flip-flops for the beach or heels for evening. A sleeveless dress will still accommodate the thicker straps on your bra.

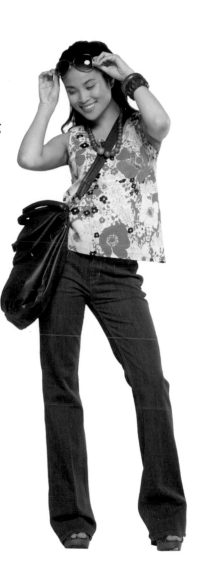

A sleeveless top shows off those slim arms.

A print top works when the fabric drapes gently over your beautiful bump!

Printy post-pregnancy

You barely need to accessorize a busy floral print top like this; just pull out one of the colours for a bag. Flared jeans are a figure-flattering option and add some funky wedge heels for leg lengthening height with added foot support!

Chic Shrug

Little tops work best when your bangers are blooming! A bright bolero or shrug like this will emphasize your shoulders, and the three-quarter sleeves draw the focus to your forearms. Dark skinny jeans will elongate that silhouette.

Back-to-work Mum

A bowling bag is
a great option for
working mums;
sling-everything-in
and it still looks
smart!

Ballet pumps look so
cool; they're smart
enough for the
office and still easy
for the school run.

twinset and trousers

For busy mums who still need to look on
it at the office, the twinset and trousers
look is a lifesaver. Comfortable enough
to get the kids off to school in, and still
smart and stylish for work – maybe you
can have it all!

School run Suit

Need to be formal for work? Simple
black trousers are perfect and they'll
slim down that belly area. A cute jacket
with its trendy neckline and sleeve detail
doesn't need anything underneath, and
the short sleeves will keep you cool.

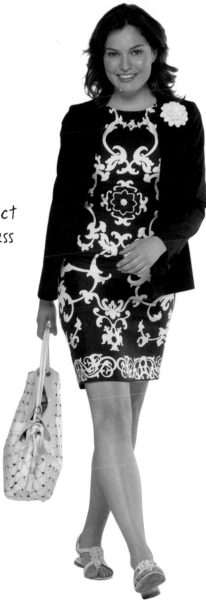

Cute corsages like this one are perfect for adding lightness to a smart black jacket.

School-run Mum

What you need right now is a bold, confident and stylish print like this one, lady! A glorious print is easy to pull off, just keep the rest of your outfit super-simple, you'll look chic and confident!

Monochrome is easy to find matching accessories for, but keep them simple with a bold print. And for an ultra-fresh look for work, try flat sandals (but check those tootsies are smart enough for work!).

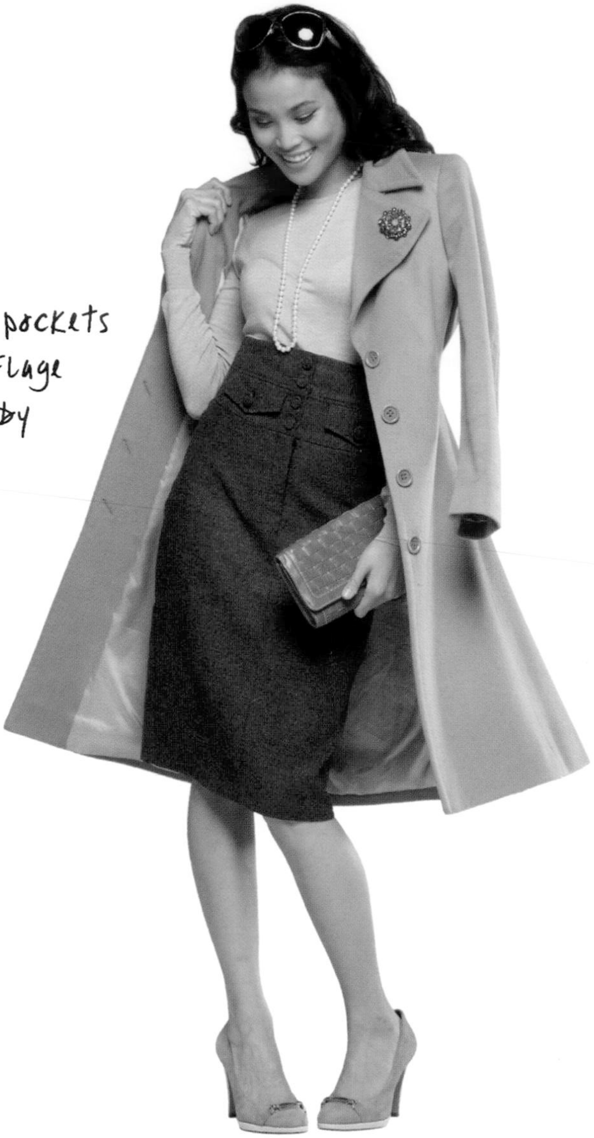

Front flap pockets
will camouflage
any post-baby
bulge.

ice Maiden Cool

This, my gorgeous, is your Grace Kelly classic glamour. If you're ever unsure about what to wear for a night out, then timelessly chic is the way to go! A single-breasted camel coat like this will never go out of style, and this high-waisted pencil skirt is a current take on a classic style and will flatter your tummy and waist. Match with oversized shades and a chic clutch bag for extra elegance.

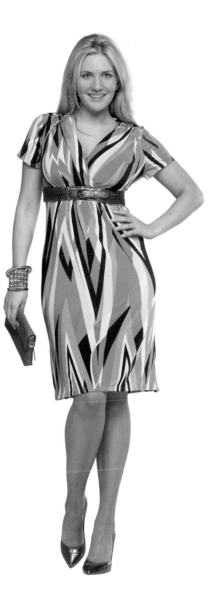

loose short sleeves like this will make your arms look slimmer than ever.

A decorative hemline shifts the focus from your tummy onto your sexy legs!

A-Line and A-List

A simple shift dress in an eye-popping colour is a great go-anywhere look for night, from bar to restaurant to nightclub. You go, girl! So if you've been out of the game, but you're now back out on the town, try a simple A-line shift to give yourself a bit of A-list style!

Bold and Beautiful

Honey, when your body confidence is a bit wobbly, go bold with a bright beautiful print! The vertical print will also help to lengthen that wider-than-usual sexy torso. And why an empire line? Because it focuses on the narrowest part of your torso: your rib cage!

Fashion-forward Mum

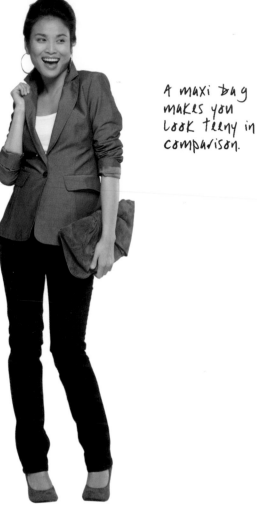

A maxi bag makes you look teeny in comparison.

A bright white top under a jacket draws the focus away from your midriff.

Foxy Tuxedo

We all know tailoring can work wonders for a girl's silhouette. So why not work the foxy tailoring look for night with a sexy tuxedo jacket? This classic style of jacket tends to be longer than the average jacket, so it covers any belly bulges. Just roll the sleeves up to show off your elegant arms.

Naughty Neckline

A bow- or tied-waist like this is perfect for disguising your pre- or post-baby bulge, and the top of this dress is genius because the double V makes it seem like you're showing off more of your rack than you actually are. (Get the same effect by wearing a V-neck top under a naughty plunging neckline!).

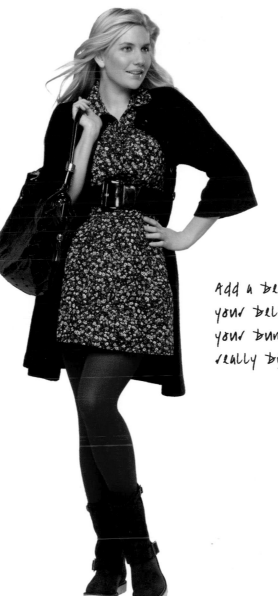

Add a belt above
your belly when
your bump gets
really big

Babe-in-boots

This sassy outfit is easy to wear, will take you anywhere and can be worn at any stage of your belly development! A loose shirtdress is smart but relaxed and a polished belt will pull your look together. A loose three-quarter-sleeve coat looks laid back but ultra-stylish. Colourful tights add an on-trend edge to this simple look.

Accessories

Rushed off your feet? Too busy to accessorize? No youtime left? Well, let Uncle Gok lighten your load. I've selected these easy accessories for you. So now the school run is your catwalk!

Pregnant

1 If you can't give up your heels when you're pregnant; ankle boots will provide extra support.

2 An eye-catching bag will distract from your bump!

3 Large earrings will keep the focus on your face, not your booty.

4 Coloured tights are a funky look and mean everyone will be looking at your lovely legs!

5   Flat slouchy boots are fashion forward and super-comfy.

6   Coloured tights are an easy and comfy way for you to keep on-trend all winter long.

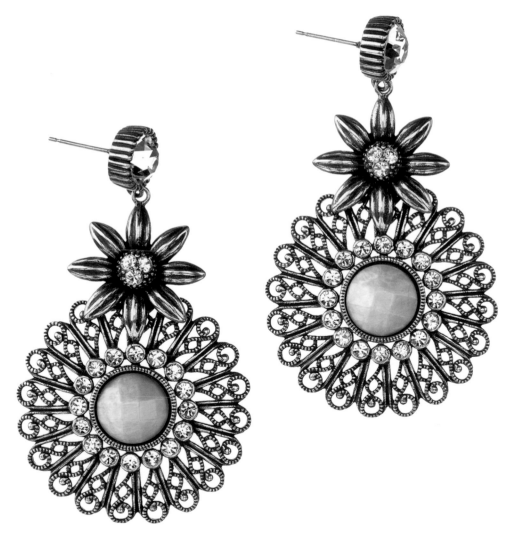

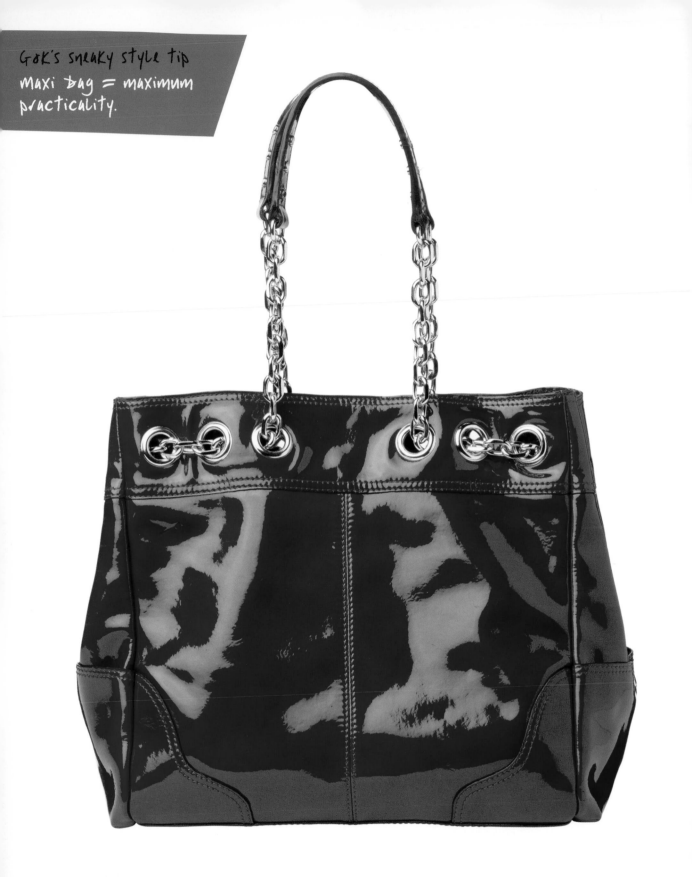

Work

1 Go for a maxi bag. They're big enough for paperwork, lip gloss and all those assorted baby things!

2 Cinch that silhouette with a contrasting belt.

3 Flat strappy sandals are chic, easy and stylish.

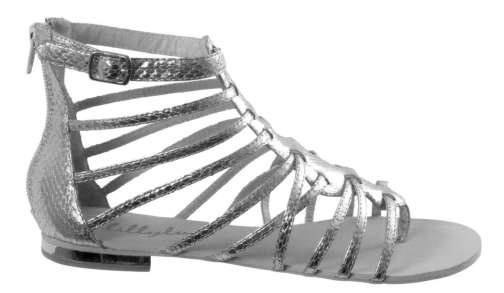

I've never understood why women are great at passing on baby clothes but hardly ever hand over their old maternity clothes. I think most women are so bored of their pregnancy wardrobes by the time they finally get back in shape they can't imagine anyone else would be interested in them. Wrong! You can never have too many maternity clothes, no matter how much they've been pre-loved. So let's recycle those jeans, share that wrap dress, lend out those riding boots, ladies!

Honey, there's no reason why your wardrobe shouldn't be just as fabulous as it's always been; it just needs some tweaking to accommodate your new routine.

Maybe there have been some changes to that fabulous figure of yours as well? Well, lady, your body is amazing and you should be proud of what it's achieved, because it's still just as gorgeous.

So, it might be a different shape or size, but girlfriend, that's as good a reason as any to invest in some new clothes. Listen to me, gorgeous – embrace the new you and let's go shopping!

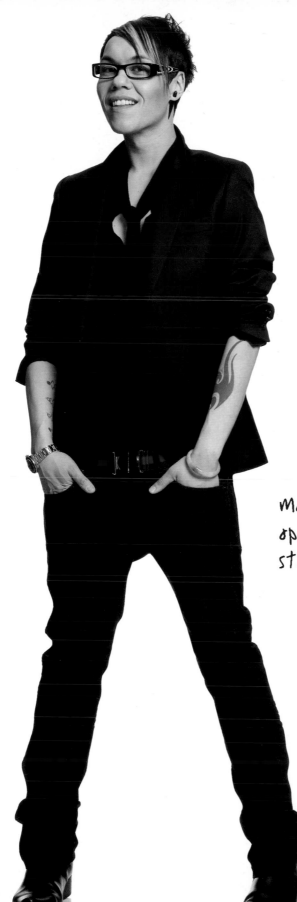

motherhood is a great opportunity for you to take stock and assess your style.

BEAUTY

Luscious lashes, effortless eyeliner and the perfect pout

- puff up your pout by dabbing high-lighter on your cupid's bow
- pinch your cheek to find your perfect shade of blusher
- always mix foundation with moisturiser

I was a make-up artist before I was a fashion stylist and I loved it. I loved making women feel great about themselves, I loved showing women how to bring out their natural beauty, and I loved playing with all the colours and brushes and products!

Make-up is fun. It's easy to get stuck into a routine once you've decided what suits you, and that's fine, because sometimes you just need to present a groomed image, fast. But you might also be losing out on looking as good as you can be. Your face, skin and colouring keep changing over the years, so the chances are, what suited you five years ago could probably do with an update!

There are loads of great tips in this chapter, but when you want to really take it to the next level, I recommend getting taught on a beauty counter. Some of those make-up-counter women can look horrendous, but professional make-up ranges, like MAC, make a point of only employing qualified make-up artists, and they can really teach you what to do.

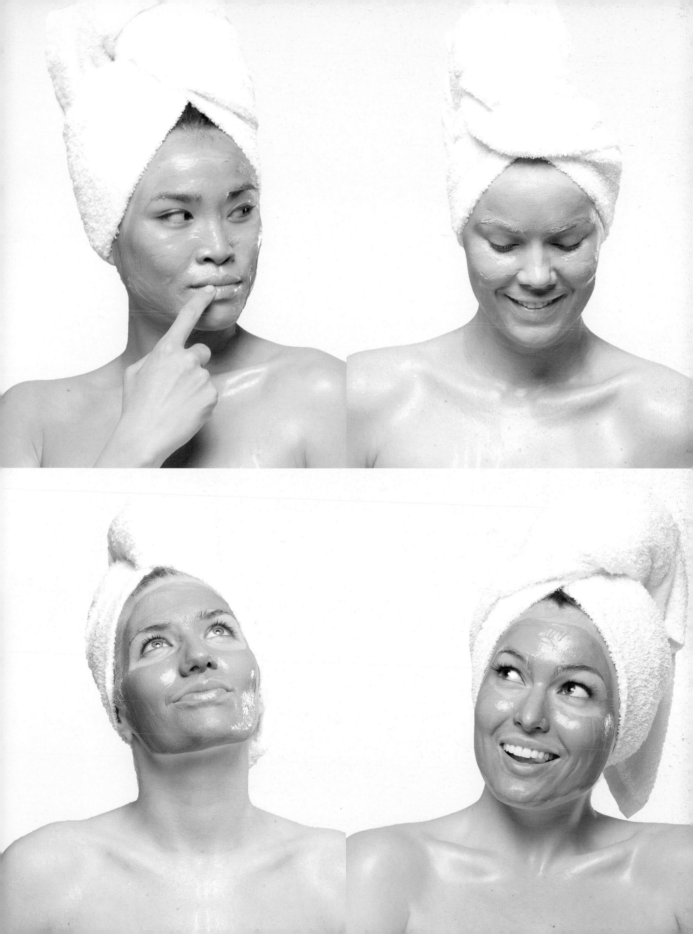

Tools

Products are great, but any make-up artist will tell you, it's more about tools than the make-up. If you can treat yourself to a good brush, or brushes, made from fine hairs, it's much easier to blend than using a cotton bud or a finger.

Preparation

I know from experience that make-up always sits better on skin that's been taken care of. I don't mean on a perfect complexion, just skin that has had a little TLC.

It's really important to find and use your perfect moisturizer. I don't think you have to spend more to get a good one; some people will only use super-expensive products like Crème de la Mer, other people swear by budget buys like Nivea. The point is to find the one that suits you.

Your skin is in its most natural state at night. While you sleep it is relaxing, breathing, away from harsh sunlight. Those 8 hours are optimum skincare hours! So it's really important to cleanse thoroughly before bed. Those facial wipes are great for taking make-up off, but they don't remove all the dirt. You need a proper cleanser to really get into the skin and take off the excess dirt. Splash with toner and cold water, and then apply a really rich night-time moisturizer.

This sounds like hard work, but when you get into a routine, its really easy, and really worth it!

In the daytime, cleanse and tone and then splash your skin with really cold water. This refreshes and wakes up your skin, and also closes pores. Apply a light day moisturizer with SPF, then allow it to absorb. Never put on your make-up without having applied a moisturizer first, it just won't sit well on the skin.

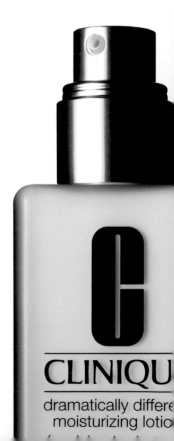

I also recommend exfoliating twice a week to remove excess skin. But avoid the harsh scrubs; you want something with granules so smooth you can barely feel them.

I don't believe in all the different products for eyes, neck and lips. A good cleanser, toner and moisturizer are all you need. But you do have to use the right products for your skin type, so if you have combination skin, you should also use an oil control moisturizer on that T-zone.

And now, your glowing skin is ready for Gok's make-up masterclasses!

Morning, beautiful – the hangover cure

With a hangover, the first thing that gets affected is your skin; it'll be all blotchy and icky, so after cleansing, start with a really good moisturizer to rehydrate your skin.

A light tinted moisturizer is essential; blend all over the face. Try using a luminescent light-reflecting concealer (the best known is YSL's Touche Eclat), and add a touch around your nose, chin and eyes to instantly take away any dark circles and redness.

So your boss really doesn't notice you've been burning the candle at both ends, add a light blusher to your skin, the same colour as your natural blush (just pinch your cheek to find your perfect shade). To get rid of the bleary eye, use white eyeliner inside the bottom rim of your eye; it'll minimize redness and make eyes appear brighter.

219

Special occasions – making an effort

For me, there are three different make-up areas: eyes, lips and skin. The trick to a great make-up look is to never mix eyes and lips; choose one or the other to highlight for your look.

Keep it simple; start with creating a flawless skin. Never use a full foundation – always mix your foundation with an equal amount of moisturizer. Then use an illuminating highlighter stick on any part of your face that sticks out; cheekbones, brow bone, down the length of your nose. This will give natural contours to your face.

Next up, blusher on those cheeks. There are three ways to apply blusher, a full line along the cheekbone, or shading underneath for contouring. And for as natural a look as possible, just smile as hard as you can and gently apply the blusher in a circular motion to the apples of your cheeks. Use a flesh-toned eye shadow over the whole lid, then apply a darker neutral shade of beige or grey colour into the outer socket.

Add clear lip gloss and mascara, and you're good to go! For more of an eveningwear or dramatic look, add kohl eyeliner along the upper lashes, and a deeper lip gloss.

New love glow – 3 dates, 3 looks

On your all important first date, you'll want to look as much like the girl next door as possible, so that it's you that shines. If you usually wear tons of eye make-up or full-on lipstick, tone down as much as possible for date No. 1.

Follow the Special Occasions beauty routine, but try adding a little subtle romantic colour – like lilac – to the eye shadow, instead of the neutral tone. For a sultry seductive finish, make sure lips are heavily glossed.

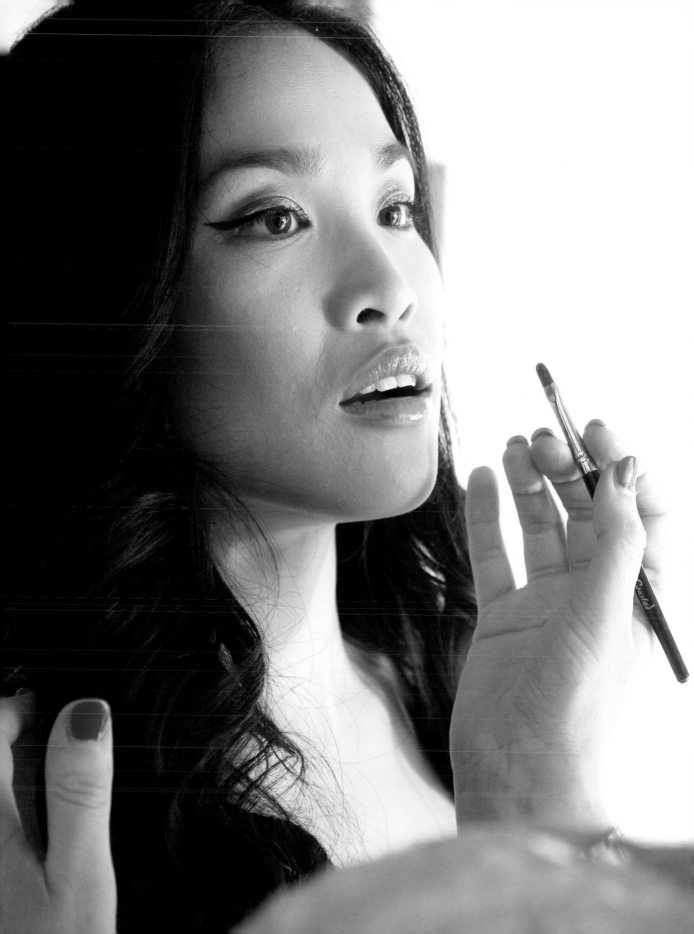

For your second date, add a slightly deeper shadow to the eyes, and a bit more mascara (prepare the lashes with an eyelash curler). Then contour the cheeks with a sweep of blusher beneath the cheekbone. A slightly more 'done' look, to keep him interested.

For your third date, I would use a natural beige or flesh-toned eye shadow. Then heavier lips. Use a lip liner to stop the lipstick from bleeding. For perfect lips, apply the lipstick, next blot with a single piece of tissue, then apply a second coat, and blot again. This takes off any excess colour, and ensures the lipstick stays in place.

Natural Beauty – you, on a good day

This is a great look: natural beauty. And you'll be amazed how pretty you can look, wearing so little make-up.

Start with a good tinted moisturizer. Brush with a light, loose translucent powder. (Or try a product like Superfix from MAC; it's a foundation in powder form with a brush, which will hold on to your tinted moisturizer).

Then comb the eyebrows through with a little mascara, and add mascara to your lashes. Apply lip gloss or lip balm and let your cheeks flush naturally.

The real key to the natural look is preparation, your eyebrows should always be plucked, but in a natural way (no harsh overplucked lines). And nobody needs to know you're wearing anything.

Speed beauty – 3 products, 3 minutes

Mums, don't think I don't know that you have about two minutes to do your make-up in the morning, if you're lucky. So, this one is for you. Forget foundation. Foundation takes all of the colour out of your face to create a clean canvas, so then you have to add all the colours and contours back in. No time!

So I'm going to keep this really simple. After you've cleansed and let your moisturizer sink in (I'm guessing you're multi-tasking at this point), just brush on some loose colourless (translucent) blotting powder with a big fluffy brush. Next add a good mascara to your lashes (mascaras work best if you replace them every couple of months; they'll go on better and quicker, so it's worth updating). Then, slick on some pink lipgloss; those Lancôme Juicy Tubes have great light colours.

So that's you, beautiful, in just three products.

Beach Beauty – looking hot in the heat

On a hot holiday, your make-up is going to change with your wardrobe. My best tip is to use a gradually tanning moisturizer for a couple of weeks before you go, including on your face (and do use a special facial gradual-tanning moisturizer on your face, they're more subtle). So you will already have a natural warmer tone when you arrive, and you will just need to add a light moisturizer with a good SPF.

Powder blusher will clog your pores in the heat, so blend in some cream blusher in a natural shade instead, which will have better staying power. A waterproof mascara will also be sweatproof. And find a lipgloss with a high SPF to protect those pretty lips.

When it comes to make-up,
you can never have too many
nifty tricks. Here are some
of my trade secrets.

Gok's sneaky tips

- Blending eyeliner is easy: just dip your blending brush in the eyeshadow that you've used, so when smudging, the eye colour blends in perfectly.

- Liquid eyeliner 'wings' are tricky to do. To get the perfect balance every time, take a measurement with the thin end of a make-up brush, and place a tiny dot at the edge of an eye for where you want the wing to end. Then match the dot on the other eye and paint on even lines. You can do the same with pencilling or powdering in an eyebrow. The point is that it's easier to take off a tiny dot than to take off a whole line.

- It can be difficult to apply lip liner without it going uneven (so you end up looking like Elvis). The best plan is to start from the bow of your lips, gradually working out on each side to get the lips even. Get a cotton bud and blend into the lips and your liner will work!

- Avoid that tide mark at all costs! Blend foundation with a sponge around your ears and neckline, to avoid a join.

- If you ever forget to take off your mascara and eye make-up after a heavy night (naughty), the best remover to use is an oil-based one. And failing that, good old Vaseline on a cotton bud is the quickest way to take it all off.

- For an instant healthy look; use a light metallic shade of eye shadow to put two little dots on the inside corner of your eyes then blend back up the lid. This lightens your face and makes your eyes look wider and more awake.

- Who doesn't want fuller lips? Puff up your pout by dabbing a tiny amount of highlighter to your cupid's bow.

SHOPPING

Beat the crowds, bargain hunting and
beyond the high street

- save time by shopping for lingerie online
- some stores still offer a personal shopping
  service during the sales
- avoid getting in a style rut by taking
  an inventory of your wardrobe

Believe me, I know how to shop! Of course, I have to do it for my job (but also I am just a total shopaholic).

Choosing outfits for my girls on the TV shows and for the celebrities I style for photo shoots is loads of fun, and it's great pulling out outfits that I know are going to totally transform someone's appearance and make their day! And for me, part of the thrill is in hunting down those special pieces.

Of course, shopping can sometimes feel like looking for a needle in a haystack. It can be frustrating and tiring and fruitless. But over the years I've learnt some sneaky tricks, short cuts and insider secrets that have helped get me out of a fashion black hole on loads of occasions.

Now, I'm going to impart my Top Ten Gok's shopping secrets (shhh; don't let anyone else know, though).

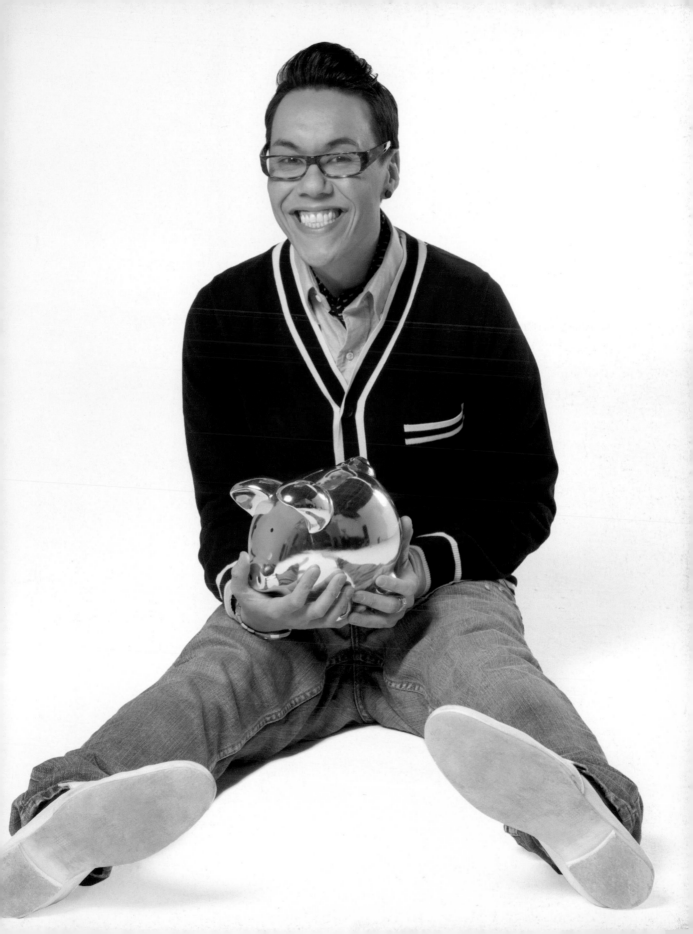

Gok's Shopping Secrets

1 Shop alone

Oh, you girls! Yes, I know it's fun to make a day of it with friends. But results-wise, this is a no-no. You know why? For the same reason that you think it's a good idea: because eeeeeeeveryone has an opinion!

The thing is, those opinions won't necessarily be the best advice! Sometimes people are biased without even realizing. Sometimes your mum doesn't want you to look like a hot foxy minx, sometimes your best friend can't get her head around you in a radical new look, sometimes your boyfriend just wants to get home for the football ('Yeah; that looks great. Let's go …').

Besides, when it comes to finding your own personal style, you have to learn to think for yourself and trust your own fashion instincts, and that's so much easier to do on your own, in your own sweet time.

And because sometimes you get the best results with a retail blitz, like trying on twelve pairs of jeans in a row. And, let's face it, no love can survive that.

2 Shop with a pro

Many stores now have personal shoppers or personal stylists (they're the same thing!). These people really know the stock and, best of all, will have it waiting for you on a rail in your own private fitting room, often bigger and posher than the usual changing rooms. Get you, A-list lady! Sometimes they even have fun perks such as free refreshments, magazines for you to read while you wait, and samples of beauty products for you to try (love that).

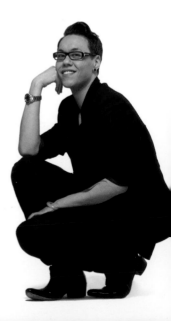

For the widest variety of styles and labels, try a department store. Where possible, ask the personal shopper to pull out some things for you before you get there, to save time. This is nearly always a complimentary service and the shoppers genuinely won't mind if you choose not to buy anything. So the only pressure you should feel under is whether you'll ever be able to go back to normal shopping (like the riffraff) again!

A good shopper will be able to help you put a cool outfit together, as well as just finding a single item. They'll also get things altered for you in-store (perfect for my unique bootied cuties who can never fit off-the-rack cuts).

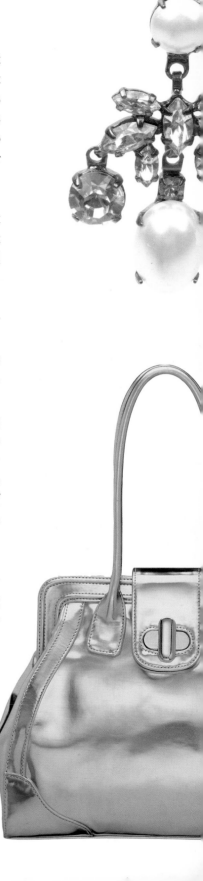

3 Shop early, shop first

It's the early bird that gets the, er, awesome strapless dip-dye prom dress. If you've never been in a shop first thing in the morning (and why would you have been?) you'd be amazed at how deserted it is. I'm not suggesting you sleep on the pavement overnight like a demented sale shopper (like I do, in front of Harvey Nichols). But as many shops restock their goodies overnight, getting there in the first couple of hours of trading seriously ups your chances of getting first grabs (I'm making this sound like an Olympic sport, aren't I?).

So shop as early as you can, especially during hideously busy times like at the weekends. Or really, really late. Some big stores shut very late in the evening, especially on a Thursday or Friday night, when most people are out on the town.

Shopping off-peak not only helps you avoid the crowding and the stress of shopping at busier times, but you will also be able to grab things before they sell out, and have the staff to yourself to search in the stockroom for that extra size or just give you some one-on-one style advice.

4 Don't get stuck in a rut

Take an inventory of your wardrobe: is it all tops? All jeans? All dresses? All purple? It's great to have a signature look, but when you have 27 tops and just one pair of jeans for them to go with, you're missing out on some great style opportunities (believe me, I know many 'top-aholics'!).

Sometimes when you go shopping, you have to be a bit strict with yourself, and not let yourself buy another black crew neck sweater. Really knowing what's in your wardrobe will help you work out what you need (see also Tip 10: Experiment Every Time).

5 Make friends in store

If you have a favourite shop, it's so worth making friends with the manager. Just a simple 'hello again' every time you make a purchase, a bit of a chat about why you love their clothes, and before you know it, she'll be warning you not to buy something because it's about to go into the sale, calling around other stores for you to find that sold-out dress, giving you a discount even though you didn't cut out that magazine coupon, or putting stuff aside for you because she knows you'll love it.

6 Find 'your' store

When you first go into a shop the number of styles can seem pretty overwhelming. But funnily enough, a lot of shops have a standard woman that they cut their clothes for. And often these seem to fit with national stereo-types, so American stores have more generous cuts, and Japanese stores are great for petites, all those Spanish stores seem to cater for tall skinny girls, and there are British stores that have dream cuts for an English pear.

You might think I'm exaggerating, and of course all stores have different sizes, different styles that will work for all their customers. But you will also find that the store where you bought your favourite pair of black trousers probably also has a pair of jeans or the perfect jacket with your name on it!

I would never encourage you to shop at just one store, but if the skirt fits …

7 Avoid the sales

Because if you didn't want it at full price … I know, I know, I'm such a party pooper! I never shop in the sales because even I go mad and make Terrible Mistakes when I do (er, purple boat shoes? What was I thinking?). And, besides, the sales are probably the most unpleasant way possible to shop, like trying to fight your way out of a clothes recycling bin.

Of course, if you tried on something earlier in the season and cried your eyes out because you couldn't afford it, and then you see it on sale – buy it! (I'm not that hard-hearted!)

There are, however, two occasions when I will make an exception:

- Some stores still offer their usual returns policy, even on sales stock. So you have a cooling-off period when you can bring back impulse buys (but always check first). So you never need have that 'what have I done?!' moment (we've all been there). And better yet, some stores will refund you the difference in price if an item you buy then gets reduced within a week.

- Some stores still offer a personal shopping service during the sales. Yes, you read that right. So while everyone else is in a rugby scrum on the shop floor, you can glide into a private fitting room with a clothes rail filled with clothes that have been pre-selected for you, in your size. Bliss.

8 Wear the right shopping outfit

I don't mean to avoid getting snooty sales assistants, like in *Pretty Woman*. I mean an outfit that doesn't take a Houdini-style contortion act to get out of every time you want to try something on. Slip on shoes, like ballet pumps, a pair of jeans and an easy to pull off top, to save you from getting into a fitting room frenzy. And don't forget your most invisible nudey seamless underwear.

And obviously, always bring anything you intend to wear with your purchase, like your killer heels, to try with it before you buy.

9 Shop online

Seriously, there is no better way – especially if you're shopping at a store you've already got clothes from so you know your sizes. But if you're unsure, stick to the sites for big name high street stores until you get the hang of it. The great thing about internet shopping is that you can do it when you've got time, and not when the shops are open – 2 in the morning with a screaming baby? Check. 11pm and waiting for a teenager to come home? Check.

Here are your top three items to look for on the web:

Lingerie

No more searching through endless numbers of bras only to find they don't have your size! Most specialist underwear shops have an online store these days.

Sales

Honey, these are a nightmare in the stores (see above – avoid at all costs!) but online it's a different story. Sale shopping on the internet doesn't involve endless rails, discarded items on the floor and, best of all, there are no other shoppers to contend with. And you can usually return sale items, but DO check.

Special items

Ever seen something in a mag, only to pop to the shops that weekend to find it's sold out? Yep, me too. But by buying online in a spare five minutes, you not only get in there before everyone else has a chance, but you might also be able to showcase that new purchase before the weekend comes.

And if you really are low tech, go mail order. Many of the big retailers still have catalogues you can leaf through at your leisure, and the same principle applies – whether it's in print or online, you're shopping to your schedule.

So grab yourself a glass of wine and settle down for some youtime. Just be careful not to drink and splurge …

10 Experiment every time

This is my top tip for developing your personal style. Every time you go into a changing room, take in one item that is so not 'you'. Whether it's a colour you never wear, a style you're convinced you'll hate, or a length of skirt that slightly frightens you! Or take a chance on something that looks rubbish on the hanger (stores know all about hanger appeal, so if they're selling it when it looks like an old rag on the hanger, it might well look brilliant on!). You may well find something you love. And if not, you've lost nothing, and will probably have made yourself laugh!

And finally … there's more to shopping than retail. Try swapping parties with friends, car-boot sales, vintage markets, borrowing stuff from your friends and family, and maybe even sewing!

Never be afraid to experiment with new looks or colours. Style is all about having fun!

Final Word

So, my gorgeouses, now you know how to wow everyone with your fabulous personal style, whatever invitations come your way! But the first date in your diary should be a naughty day of shopping for the new style-savvy you. I know you're going to come up with some amazing looks, and have lots of fun along the way. I'm so proud of you! This book will always provide some one-on-one styling advice, so come back to it whenever you're having a fashion dilemma. Now get out there and flaunt those foxy outfits!

And remember, Gok says ... you deserve to look fabulous every day!

Gok
X

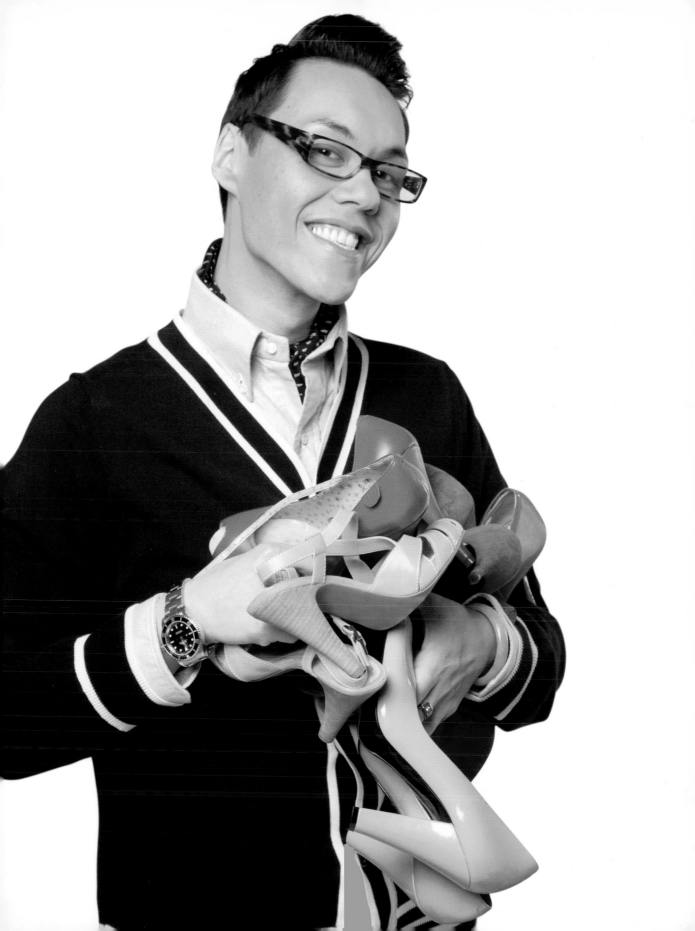

notes

notes

notes

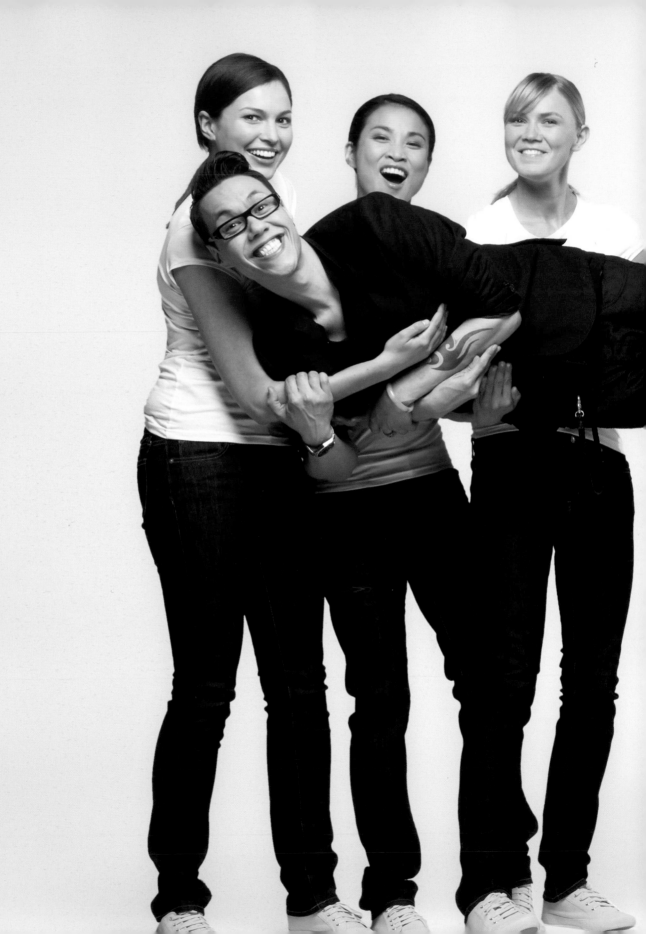

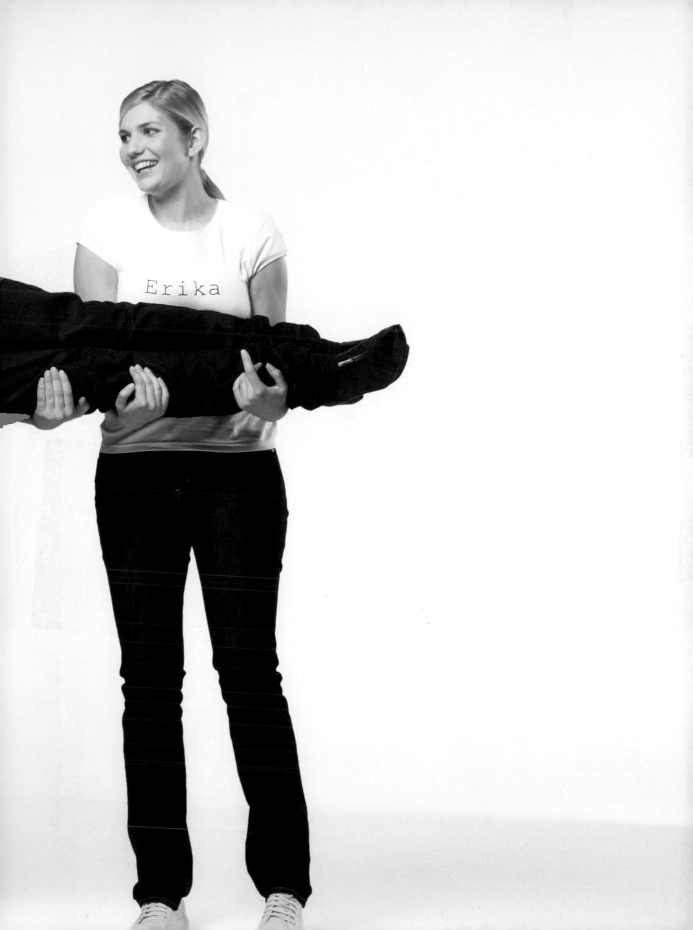

Acknowledgements

Firstly, I want to say a huge thank you to my family, who have continued to support me and give me time away from them, even when I was most needed. In particular my Mum, whose night-time calls when I am most exhausted have reminded me of just how loved I am. A special set of kisses to the most beautiful girls in the world, Maya Lily and Lola Rose. May you both grow to be honest, kind and beautiful, inside and out. Uncle Gok loves you both dearly!

To all my fabulous friends who have allowed me to go AWOL but have embraced me, without exception, on my return.

A huge thank you to my Jewish Mum who manages my time, diary and moods so efficiently, even though she has a family of her own.

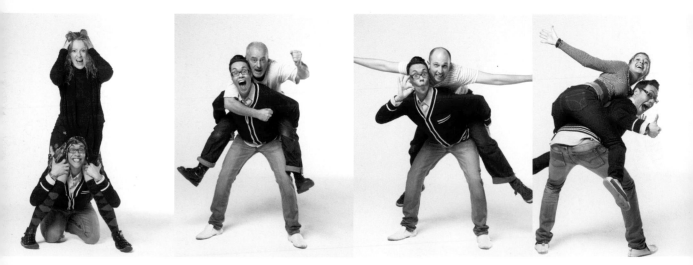

A big thank you to Channel 4, and especially to Sue Murphy for all your commitment and guidance and, most of all, your friendship.

To everyone at 'Barkers' Harpers for your patience, support and guidance.

To Angela for the coffee, pap shots and sheer fashion brilliance that you have brought to this book.

To the models and crew involved in producing the book, in particular to Kirsty – without her the shots would never have been shot!

To all of you who buy this book, may you never have another day badly dressed! Vive La Femme!!!!

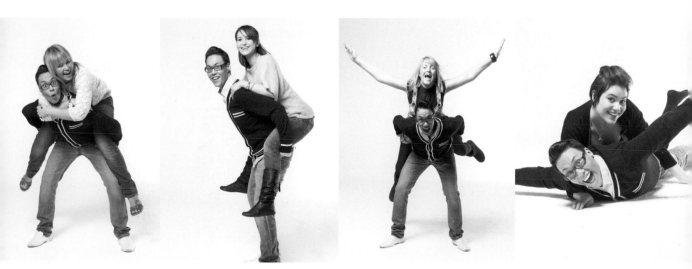

Directory

A huge thank you to all the shops who supplied us with their lovely clothes. Here's where they came from.

Basics

p.15 Red bra, Gossard; boy shorts, Topshop; red patent stilettos, Pied à Terre; model, Cat

pp.19 and 21 Slouchy jersey top, Reiss; cream trousers, Simply Be; grey scarf used as headband, Jaeger; hoop earrings, Accessorize; clutch bag, Accessorize; peep-toe grey shoes, H&M; model, Trese-San

p.20 Brown jersey sleeveless dress, Banana Republic; cream pashmina, Gap; brown woven bag, Miss Sixty; brown high heels, Strutt Couture; bangles, Angie Gooderham; necklace, Angie Gooderham; model, Bailee

p.22 Jacket, Jaeger; grey jumper, Phase Eight; houndstooth check skirt, New Look; socks, H&M; black shoes, Red or Dead; felt beenie and patent bow belt, Sara Berman; model, Trese-San

p.23 Top, H&M; jeans, H&M; flat sandals, Gap; model, Bailee

p.24 Brown tweed batwing coat, Dorothy Perkins; large gem brooch, Banana Republic; tights, Topshop; dark brown leather boots, Kew; mini tan leather bag, Kew; model, Trese-San

p.25 left Grey polo neck, Phase Eight; light grey jersey t-shirt, Reiss; blue denim shorts, Century 21; grey knee-length socks, H&M; flat brogues, Ted Baker; grey trilby hat, Kangol; necklaces, Freedom at Topshop; patchwork clutch bag, Topshop; black-rimmed glasses, Giorgio Armani at Safilo; model, Cat

p.25 right Brown, black and orange jersey wrap-effect dress, Fenn Wright Mason at House of Fraser; biscuit-coloured polo neck, John Smedley; tan leather boots, Kew; brown leather bag, John Lewis; striped socks, H&M; orange disc necklace, Diva at Miss Selfridge; model, Erica

p.26 Chunky navy cardigan, Phase Eight; floral dress, River Island; brown leather belt, Sara Berman; brown mini leather satchel, Warehouse; brown wedges, River Island; socks, H&M; model, Bailee

p.27 Blue blouse, Banana Republic; blue cardigan, TSEsay; dark blue knee-length skirt, Gap; wide purple leather belt, Topshop; multicoloured bead necklace, Freedom at Topshop; navy blue leather bag, Hayley Anna; knee-length socks, H&M; silver court shoes, Office; model, Cat

p.28 left Grey knitted dress, Phase Eight; black leather jacket, Topshop; black tights, Falke; yellow patent ballet pumps, Russell & Bromley; yellow and black clutch bag, Topshop; model, Erica

p.28 right Beige trench coat, Principles; dark brown leather boots, Kew; brown leather satchel bag, Warehouse; multicoloured scarf, stylist's own; model, Erica

p.29 left Blue blazer with badge, Kate Moss at Topshop; white shirt, Jaspar Conran; white skinny trousers, Gap; black skinny belt, Jesiré; gold ballet pumps, Topshop; sunglasses, Banana Republic; bag, Warehouse; neckscarf, stylist's own; model, Cat

pp.29 right and 109 Tan leather jacket, Tommy Hilfiger; straight-leg jeans, Gap; brown wedges, River Island; white-rimmed sunglasses, Carrera by Safilo; large tan leather bag, Tommy Hilfiger; bangles, Accessorize; scarf worn as head scarf, stylist's own; model, Bailee

p.30 Black and white striped vest top, Jasper Conran at Debenhams; faded blue jeans, 7 For All Mankind at John Lewis; ballet pumps, Jones the Bootmakers; pink scarf, Topshop; model, Erica

p.31 left Vest top, Topshop; blue sailor front jeans, Topshop; ballet pumps, Russell & Bromley; model, Trese-San

p.31 right Spotty vest top, Joules; skinny striped jeans, Razor Office; pumps, Ted Baker; model, Cat

p.32 Brown riding boots, River Island

p.33 Giant pave ball ring, Accessorize

p.34 Clear bead necklace, Dorothy Perkins

p.35 Multicoloured Mary Jane shoes, Faith

Underwear

pp.41 and 54 Grey and olive frilly bra and knickers, Huit at Figleaves; nude hold-ups, H&M; nude patent round-toe shoes, LK Bennett; model, Trese-San

pp.43 and 52 Red satin corset, Simply Yours; black frilly knickers with suspenders, Ann Summers; black fishnet stockings, Agent Provocateur; black high-heel shoes, Red or Dead; flower, Freedom at Topshop; model, Bailee

pp.45 and 59 Knitted shawl, Dorothy Perkins; nude bra, Bodas; printed boy shorts, Topshop; knitted ankle socks, Topshop; model, Trese-San

pp.47 and 61 right Pale pink ruched bra and knickers, Knickerbox; pink knitted shrug, Topshop; pink and black ballet pumps, Russell & Bromley; model, Cat

p.48 Nude bra, Simply Yours; nude high-waisted control pants, Spanx; sleeveless cardigan, Principles; model, Erica

p.49 Nude bra, Just Peachy at Figleaves; nude waister, Miraclesuit at Figleaves; half shorts, Spanx; model, Bailee

p.50 left Black push-up bra, Shapely Figures at Simply Be; high-waisted control pants, Marks & Spencer; snakeskin peep-toe shoes, Aldo; model, Bailee

p.50 right Black bodysuit, Spanx; black high-heel shoes, Aldo; black fishnet scarf, stylist's own; model, Erica

p.51 Ivory and black lace camisole and knickers, Rigby & Peller; black stockings, Love Kylie Legs at Figleaves; black peep-toe heels with pompom, Red or Dead; mini top hat, stylist's own; model, Trese-San

p.53 Red corset, Ann Summers; black knickers, Ann Summers; stockings, Love Kylie Legs at Figleaves; black high-heel shoes, Aldo; cuffs, Ann Summers; model, Bailee

p.55 Pink polka-dot knickers and bra, Star by Julien Macdonald at Debenhams; black peep-toes with pompoms, Red or Dead; model, Erica

p.56 Pink-striped bra and knicker set, La Senza; blue socks, H&M; floral short-sleeve shirt, CCL; model, Cat

p.57 Pink camisole with bra and suspenders, Star by Julien Macdonald at Debenhams; stockings, John Lewis; nude shoes, Reiss; model, Erica

p.58 Printed vest and thong set, Tommy Hilfiger; grey cardigan, Republic; argyle socks, Burlington at John Lewis; model, Trese-San

p.60 Black and cream lace bra and knickers, Knickerbox; long grey cardigan, Phase Eight; grey scarf, Jaeger; red socks, H&M; model, Cat

p.61 left Purple chiffon bra and knickers, SPANKS at Figleaves; white shirt, Formes; model, Cat

p.63 Brown chiffon shrug, vintage

p.64 Plum long leather gloves, Hobbs

p.65 Black peep-toe shoes, Dune

Workwear

pp.71 and 83 Black skirt with horizontal stripes and bow, Warehouse; black satin and chiffon shirt, Principles; brown leather bag, John Lewis; brown patchwork shoes, Kate Kuba; flower, Freedom at Topshop; earrings, stylist's own; model, Trese-San

p.73 Pussy-bow blouse, Miss Selfridge; pencil skirt, Alexander McQueen at Selfridges; suede court shoes, Christian Louboutin; glasses, Specsavers; model, Trese-San

p.78 Red sleeveless shift dress, Jesiré; white patent belt, Zara; black tights, Falke; black necklace, Angie Gooderham; sunglasses, Christian Dior by Safilo; black shoes, Aldo; handbag, Oasis; model, Bailee

p.79 Beige safari-style sleeveless dress and belt, Star by Julien Macdonald at Debenhams; brown shoes, Brantano; large green shopper bag, Topshop; necklace, Wallis; bangles, Angie Gooderham and Accessorize; multicoloured headscarf, Freedom at Topshop; model, Erica

p.80 Knee-length high-waisted grey skirt, River Island; white frilly sleeveless blouse, New Look; black leather belt, LK Bennett; trilby, Kangol; grey peep-toe shoes, H&M; bag, Faith; model, Erica

p.81 Charcoal trousers, Wallis; white short-sleeve shirt, Tommy Hilfiger; grey waistcoat, Debenhams; trilby hat, M&S; black leather gloves, Dents; flat black shoes, Jones; model, Erica

p.82 left Black high-waisted trousers, River Island; leopard-print pussy-bow blouse, Miss Selfridge; black leather belt, LK Bennett; black flat pointy pumps, Jones; black leather structured bag, Cross at Selfridges; earrings, Accessorize; model, Cat

p.82 right Red, black and white swirl pattern wrap dress, Phase Eight; white patent belt, Zara; black egg necklace, Angie Gooderham; black tights, Jonathan Aston; black and white court shoes, Faith; model, Erica

p.84 Grey suit, Hugo Boss; red t-shirt, TSE; grey peep-toe shoes, H&M; black structured leather bag, Cross at Selfridges; handbag, Banana Republic; sunglasses, Alexander McQueen by Safilo; model, Bailee

p.85 left Grey crew-neck top, John Smedley; grey wool dress with sequins (worn over polo neck), Phase Eight; red cardigan, John Smedley; black belt, LK Bennett; white patent structured bag, LK Bennett; bracelet, New Look; pearl necklace, Pilgrim; grey Mary Jane shoes, Warehouse; model, Trese-San

p.85 right Black pinstripe shift dress and suit jacket, Jaeger; grey shirt, Preen; black tie, Topman; black tights, Falke; multicoloured Mary Jane shoes, Faith; model, Cat

p.86 left Purple bouclé jacket and skirt, New Look; frilly cream shirt, Topshop; black elasticated belt, Topshop; burgundy tights, Falke; black patent ankle boots, Kate Kuba; bag, Russell & Bromley; model, Bailee

p.86 right White short-sleeve shirt, Tommy Hilfiger; purple skinny trousers, H&M; red belt, Uniqlo; red leather stilettos, Pied à Terre; clutch bag, Warehouse; model, Trese-San

p.87 White t-shirt, Primark; green cardigan, Banana Republic; black trousers and belt, River Island; woven straw bag with chain, Topshop; white sneakers, Topshop; accessories, stylist's own; model, Trese-San

p.88 Textured circle bracelet, QVC

p.89 Pink and black shoe boots, Moda in Pelle

p.90 Black fringed bag, Jaeger

p.91 Beaded bracelet, Angie Gooderham

Going Out

pp.101 and 113 Blue sleeveless flapper dress with beading and fringing, River Island; clutch bag, Oasis; flower, Freedom at Topshop; silver and Perspex sandals with diamanté detail on strap, Stuart Weitzman; model Trese-San

pp.103 and 109 Lilac tiered dress, Topshop; hot pink bolero shrug, Coast; black leather belt, Topshop; shoes, Schuh; flower, Barnett Lawson; model, Trese-San

pp.105 and 112 Green and black strapless dress, Felder & Felder at Selfridges; long black leather gloves, Dents; bag, Russell & Bromley; ring, Accessorize; black shoes, Aldo; model, Trese-San

p.106 Black and silver sleeveless dress, Star by Julien Macdonald at Debenhams; black bead and flower bracelet, Freedom at Topshop; black clutch bag, Banana Republic; black tights, Topshop; black high heels, Red or Dead; model, Erica

p.107 Dress and belt, Warehouse; pearl necklace, Pilgrim; pearl bracelet, New Look; gloves and clutch bag, Dents; shoes, Red or Dead; model, Bailee

p.108 Blue v-neck mini dress, TSE; burgundy tights, Falke; pink clutch bag, Topshop; green platform shoes with wood and Perspex heel, Topshop; bangle, Freedom at Topshop; model, Erica

p.110 left Skinny blue jeans, Uniqlo; heavy sequin cream tank top, Debenhams; small clutch bag, Oasis; earrings, Warehouse; cut-out grey lace-up shoes, Topshop; model, Cat

p.110 right Black silk halterneck jumpsuit, TSEsay; wide black leather belt with gold studs, Topshop; gold woven bracelet, Lara Bohinc; metallic clutch bag, Warehouse; gold and black shoes, Oasis; model, Cat

p.111 Vest top, Pringle 1815; sequin bolero, Kate Moss at Topshop; skinny jeans, Warehouse; flat silver lace-up brogues, Ted Baker; trilby, Kangol; necklace, Accessorize; earrings, Freedom at Topshop; clutch bag, Topshop; model, Bailee

p.114 left Dress, Coast; silver sequin cape, Kate Moss at Topshop; belt, Topshop; shoes, Oasis; clutch bag, Warehouse; ring and earrings, Accessorize; model, Bailee

p.114 right Long cream silk fishtail dress, Principles; white patent belt, Zara; three-pearl earrings and matching bracelet, New Look; shoes, Russell & Bromley; cream clutch bag with chain, AC Company PLL; model, Cat

p.115 Printed dress, Star by Julien MacDonald at Debenhams; flower, Topshop; silk pashmina, John Lewis; beaded purse, Accessorize; jewelled sandals, Faith; model Erica

p.117 Red patent shoes, Carvela

p.118 Vintage chiffon and sequin capelet

p.119 Pearl necklace, Mikey

Holidays

pp.127, 137 and 138 left White bikini with rainbow pattern, Topshop; mini denim shorts, Gold by Giles Deacon at New Look; bracelet, Freedom at Topshop; bag, Topshop; sunglasses, stylist's own; model, Cat

pp.129 and 146 right White t-shirt, Tommy Hilfiger; camel-coloured trousers, Banana Republic; small brown leather satchel (turned into a bumbag), Warehouse; black jumper, John Smedley; flip-flops, New Look; model, Cat

pp.131 and 140 White kaftan, Rigby & Peller; straw bag with chain handle, Topshop; bangle and ring, Lara Bohinc; headband, Freedom at Topshop; gold sandals, Schuh; model, Erica

pp.133 and 146 Blue bikini, Seafolly; long floral silk skirt, Banana Republic; wide brim hat, Kangol; large blue leather bag, Hayley Anna; multicoloured necklace, Freedom at Topshop; sunglasses, Alexander McQueen by Safilo; shoes, Brantano; bangle, Accessorize; model, Cat

p.138 right Blue tankini with brown print, Seafolly; grey-fringed bag, New Look; flat sandals, Gap; straw floppy hat, Seafolly; sunglasses, Banana Republic; model, Cat

p.139 left Hot pink swimming costume, Lisa Ho at Rigby & Peller; sunglasses, Hugo Boss by Safilo; gold necklace, Accessorize; earrings, Freedom by Topshop; gold bangles, Angie Gooderham; sandals, Schuh; gold skinny belt, stylist's own; model, Erica

p.139 right One-piece swimming costume, Sunseeker Australia; raffia and silk wedges, Russell & Bromley; earrings, Freedom at Topshop; gold woven bracelet, Lara Bohinc; sunglasses, Hugo Boss by Safilo; model, Trese-San

p.141 Printed bikini, Tommy Hilfiger; chiffon cream blouse with circular details, Nougat at House of Fraser; necklace, Accessorize; flat sandals, New Look; ribbon, stylist's own; model, Trese-San

p.142 Bikini, Seafolly; sarong, Tommy Hilfiger; bag, Topshop; earrings, Freedom at Topshop; sandals, Schuh; bangles, Angie Gooderham; model, Cat

p.143 Spotted sarong, Topshop; Bikini, Tommy Hilfiger; thong sandals, Schuh; gold bangles, Angie Gooderham; beach bag, Accessorise

p.144 Dress, Tommy Hilfiger; hat, Topshop; sunglasses, Giorgio Armani by Safilo; brown wedge sandals, River Island; large bag, Warehouse; cotton scarf, Hilfiger Denim; model, Bailee

p.145 Blue tropical-print long dress, H&M; long glass bead and chain necklace, Wallis; bangles, Accessorize; tan soft leather handbag, Hayley Anna; shoes, stylist's own; headwrap, stylist's own; model Erica

p.146 left White and black stripe vest top, Gold by Giles Deacon at New Look; black silk shorts, Pringle of Scotland; raffia and silk shoes, Russell & Bromley; scarf, Banana Republic; clutch bag, Dents; bracelets, Angie Gooderham; model, Trese-San

p.147 Multicoloured floral bandeau top, Warehouse; denim shorts, Gold by Giles Deacon at New Look; white-framed sunglasses, Carrera by Safilo; gold hoop earrings, Freedom at Topshop; white handbag, Russell & Bromley; metalic sandals, Gap; model, Trese-San

p.148 left Pink and white silk mini dress, New Look; necklace, Tatty Divine; woven clutch bag with chain, Miss Sixty; ring, Freedom at Topshop; gladiator sandals, Kurt Geiger; model, Cat

p.148 right Blue straight-leg jeans, Uniqlo; top, Topshop; earrings, Freedom at Topshop; bangles, Accessorize; shoes, Aldo; bag, Jasper Conran at Debenhams; model, Erica

p.149 Long pink and black silk dress, New Look; necklace and bangles, River Island; black frilled satin bag, Coast; jewelled thongs, Faith; model, Bailee

p.150 Nude flip-flops, Havaianas

p.151 Belly chain, stylist's own

p.152 Hexagonal gold clutch, Monsoon

p.153 Multi-coloured headscarf, stylist's own

Weddings

pp.161 and 168 Green two-piece skirt suit, Jaeger; leopard-print hat, Diva Blue; large tan leather bag, Tommy Hilfiger; tights, Marks & Spencer; gold pointy shoes, Strutt Couture; brooch, Banana Republic; model, Trese-San

pp.165 and 177 Dress, Wallis; feathered hat, Philip Somerville; nude and brown-trim ballet pumps, Banana Republic; cream pashmina, Gap; bracelets, Miss Selfridge; necklace, Freedom at Topshop; satin clutch bag, Coast; model, Bailee

pp.167 and 170 left Black and white dress with buttons, River Island; cream tights, Falke; cream hat with feather, Philip Somerville; bag, Jaspar Conran at Debenhams; nude Mary Jane shoes, Topshop; model, Trese-San

p.169 Oyster satin dress, Coast; red felt cropped coat, TSE; large black hat, Philip Somerville; opaque tights, Jonathan Aston; long purple gloves, Dents; bag, Dents; shoes, Red or Dead; model, Bailee

p.170 right Blue-patterned silk halterneck dress, Banana Republic; blue trench coat, Reiss; belt, Reiss; shoes, Strutt Couture; hat, Diva Blue; bag, Topshop; model, Bailee

p.171 Purple sleeveless dress, LK Bennett; bag, Topshop; hat, Kangol; stockings, H&M; bracelet, Freedom; shoes, Schuh; model, Erica

p.172 left Blue silk dress, Topshop; grey cardigan, Banana Republic; burgundy tights, Falke; headdress, Diva Blue; grey Mary Jane shoes, Warehouse; clutch bag, Topshop; blue leather gloves, stylist's own; model, Cat

p.172 right Coral dress, Principles; cream jacket, Phase Eight; cream hat, Debenhams; black satin floral clutch bag, Coast; nude Mary Jane shoes, Topshop; model Erica

p.173 Blue bell-sleeve cropped jacket and white t-shirt, Banana Republic; blue, green and white printed bell skirt, H&M; tights, Topshop; black shoes, Red or Dead; small black sequin hat, Philip Somerville; model, Cat

p.174 White pinstripe trouser suit, Wallis; grey skinny belt, Reiss; sunglasses, Hugo Boss by Safilo; clutch bag, Topshop; earrings, TU at Sainsbury's; grey peep-toe shoes, H&M; model, Trese-San

p.175 Black suit jacket, Wallis; black suit trousers, Anna Scholz; gold camisole, Fenn Wright Mason; black sequin hat with black quills, Diva Blue; brooch, Banana Republic; shoes, Office; bag, stylist's own; model, Erica

p.176 Cream and gold brocade sleeveless dress and belt, River Island; black feathered hat, Philip Somerville; decorative gloves, Dents; black silk floral clutch bag, Coast; earrings, Angie Gooderham; black shoes, Aldo; model, Trese-San

p.178 Mint-green flapper dress, Wallis; hat with quill, John Lewis; white patent structured bag, LK Bennett; black shoes with two straps, LK Bennett; model, Cat

p.179 Pink satin sleeveless dress with bow, Karen Millen; cream pashmina, Gap; cream hat, Debenhams; nude patent shoes, LK Bennett; small cream clutch bag, Accompany PLC; model, Erica

p.180 Beige, pink and black striped cropped jacket, Malene Birger; gold top, Fenn Wright Mason; beige fitted trousers, Gap; oversized white leather clutch bag, Hayley Anna; sunglasses, Valentino by Safilo; cream trilby, Kangol; beige patent sandals, Russell & Bromley; flower, stylist's own; model, Cat

p.181 Cream and gold cropped jacket, Pringle 1815; green skirt, Principles; cream bag, Reiss; dragonfly brooch, Angie Gooderham; red snakeskin sling-back shoes, Strutt Couture; red flower as brooch, stylist's own; model, Bailee

p.182 Hairpiece, Star by Julian Macdonald at Debenhams

p.183 Grey felt trilby, Jaeger

p.184 Two-tone patent Mary Janes, Carvela

p.185 Red leather driving gloves, Dents

Mums

p.198 left Black leather jacket, Topshop; black top, Formes; black ribbed-waist pencil skirt, Formes; black trilby, Kangol; fishnet tights, La Senza; black and yellow clutch bag, Topshop; patent ankle boots, Russell & Bromley; model, Cat

p.198 right Suit, Formes; black sandals with jewels on the strap, Blocx Emilio Luca; bag, Warehouse; dragonfly brooch, Banana Republic; model, Cat

p.199 Pink and orange chiffon sleeveless empire-line dress, Formes; necklace and bracelet, Wallis; bracelet, Accessorize; flat gold sandals, New Look; model, Cat

p.200 left Green and white sleeveless top, Mamas & Papas; jeans, Formes; yellow sun hat, Topshop; yellow ballet pumps, Russell & Bromley; multi-coloured necklace, Freedom at Topshop; bangles, Freedom at Topshop; model, Cat

p.200 right Multicoloured sleeveless dress, Phase Eight; brown fringed bag, New Look; bangles, Freedom at Topshop; black sandals, stylist's own; model, Trese-San

p.201 left Orange and white strapless top, Topshop; blue jeans, Gap; wedge sandals, River Island; large blue leather bag, Hayley Anna; sunglasses, Giorgio Armani by Safilo; necklace, Wallis; model, Trese-San

p.201 right Coral shrug, Coast; patterned dress, John Rocha at Debenhams; jeans, Uniqlo; brown croc bag and ballet pumps, LK Bennett; model, Erica

p.202 left Pink fine-knit cardigan, black flower, Freedom at Topshop; wide-leg grey trousers, Jaeger; black skinny belt, Mango; black oversize bag, Warehouse; flat black ballet pumps, Jones the Bootmaker; model, Cat

p.202 right Check fitted jacket, PC Clothing at Topshop; trousers, Jasper Conran at Debenhams; ballet pumps, Jones the Bootmakers; patent bag, Russell & Bromley; model, Trese-San

p.203 Dress, Banana Republic; coat, Reiss; shoes, Zara; bag, LK Bennett; flower, Freedom at Topshop; model, Bailee

p.204 Camel coat, Jaeger; cream fine-knit jumper, John Smedley; long high-waisted skirt, Dorothy Perkins; pearl necklace, Pilgrim; jewelled brooch, Angie Gooderham; sunglasses, Giorgio Armani by Safilo; brown clutch bag, Warehouse; nude court shoes, Banana Republic; model, Trese-San

p.205 left Pink sleeveless shift dress with flowers and jewels on hemline, DKNY; black tights, Falke; black high heels, Red or Dead; black clutch bag, Russell & Bromley; model, Cat

p.205 right White, orange and black print dress and belt, Star by Julien Macdonald at Debenhams; brown clutch bag, Warehouse; gold heels, Strutt Couture; bangles, Angie Gooderham; model, Erica

p.206 left Grey blazer, Reiss; white t-shirt, Primark; blue jeans, Gap; red shoes, Schuh; clutch bag, Topshop; model, Trese-San

p.206 right Multicoloured floral print sleeveless dress, Phase Eight; cream shoulder bag, Reiss; nude square-toe court shoes, LK Bennett; model, Bailee

p.207 Floral dress, Primark; chunky black cardigan, Red Herring at Debenhams; black belt, Topshop; black biker boots, Redwing; coloured tights, Falke; model, Erica

p.209 Earrings, Erickon Beamon at Debenhams
p.210 Red patent bag, Jaeger
p.211 Gladiator sandals, Faith

Beauty

p.218 Dramaticaly Different Moisturizing Lotion, Clinique
p.219 White eye definer, The Body Shop
p.222 Lip liners, The Body Shop

Shopping

p.231 Pearl earrings, Angie Gooderham
p.233 Pink shoe, Stuart Weitzman
p.234 Embellished leather belt, Dorothy Perkins
p.235 Black peep-toe shoes, Carvela

Beginning/end of chapter shots

pp.2, 124 and 135 Straw sunhat and cutaway swimsuit, Seafolly; sunglasses, Dior by Safilo; striped beach bag, Accessorize; bangles, Miss Selfridge and Dorothy Perkins; sandals, Stuart Weitzman at Russell & Bromley; model, Erica

p.99 from left to right Black dress, Karen Millen; jewelled clutch bag, Russell & Bromley; model, Erica. Pink ruffle dress, Reiss; diamanté trimmed leather gloves, Dents; model, Cat. Floral bolero, Coast; brocade dress, D&G at Selfridges; model, Trese-San. Dress, Temperley at Selfridges; flower, Topshop; model, Bailee

p.158 from left to right Coat and dress, Phase Eight; hat, Coast; model, Bailee. Cream chiffon shrug, Coast; cream striped dress, John Rocha at Debenhams; butterfly necklace, New Look; model, Erica. Cream and gold brocade belted dress, River Island; lilac leather gloves, Dents; cream patent peep-toe shoes, Aldo; model, Trese-San. Oyster satin dress, Coast; floral hairclip, Freedom at Topshop; cream multi-floral bouquet, Kenneth Turner; model, Cat

p.191 Orange satin dress, Reiss; black feather-trim hat, Debenhams; black patent bow belt, Sara Berman; leather gloves, Dents; patent stilettos, Aldo; model, Bailee

p.217 Towels, Christy